Arthritis

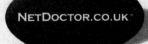

Series Editor
Dr Dan Rutherford

Hodder & Stoughton
LONDON SYDNEY AUCKLAND

First published in Great Britain in 2003

10 9 8 7 6 5 4 3 2 1

British Library Cataloguing in Publication Data
A record for this book is available from the British Library

ISBN 0 340 78687 6

Typeset in Garamond by Avon DataSet Ltd,
Bidford-on-Avon, Warwickshire

Printed and bound in Great Britain by
Bookmarque Ltd., Croydon, Surrey

The paper and board used in this paperback are natural recyclable
products made from wood grown in sustainable forests.
The manufacturing processes conform to the environmental
regulations of the country of origin.

Hodder & Stoughton
A Division of Hodder Headline Ltd
338 Euston Road
London NW1 3BH
www.madaboutbooks.com

Contents

Foreword

Arthritis and other rheumatic disorders are among the most frequent causes of ill health and disability in the population. They range from short-lived, minor aches and pains to serious, progressively disabling long-term conditions. Rarely, they can be life-threatening.

People are rightly becoming increasingly interested in health matters. They want to know how to keep well but they also want to know more about illnesses and how they should best be treated. Media channels provide a constant stream of news about advances in medical diagnosis and treatment. Rheumatology itself is advancing with ever new diagnostic techniques and more promising treatment for rheumatoid arthritis, such as the tumour necrosis factor antagonist drugs that are mentioned here. Surgery is striding forwards with more benefits for patients and consequent reduction in disability. Yet on the ground the standards of care experienced by people with joint disease can vary greatly around the country.

The NHS is changing towards more public engagement in the service it delivers. The 'Expert Patient' is an idea strongly supported by government. Our own 'Patient Carer' project in South Manchester has shown clearly that there are great benefits to be had when people are provided with good information on their illness and are given the opportunity to become involved in their own care.

The goal of the 'Help Yourself to Health' book series is to create the best contemporary medical knowledge in a style that is educational and understandable by the widest possible audience. In this volume specific aspects of arthritis and other rheumatic diseases are presented in a self-contained and comprehensive manner, linking the relevant basic scientific aspects to the condition as experienced by the patient. Up-to-date medical treatments are explained as well as their pitfalls, and how to minimise them. Many practical points will be useful to arthritis sufferers and there are references to further detailed information as well as to patient organisations and other helpful bodies. I believe this book will help the person with arthritis to be fully motivated and well informed, clearing the path for him or her to be in partnership with doctors and carers for the maximum benefit.

The World Health Organisation has designated the years 2000–2010 as the decade for arthritis and bone disorders and it has been a great pleasure for me to contribute to such a timely publication. I believe it deserves wide reading by patients, carers and families involved, directly or indirectly, with arthritis.

Dr Badal Pal MD, FRCP, D.Med Rehab
Consultant Rheumatologist and Honorary Lecturer
University of Manchester
e-mail: badal.pal@smuht.nwest.nhs.uk

Acknowledgements

There are far too few specialists in rheumatology in the UK and those we have need to work long hours to see everyone who needs their attention. Despite many other demands Dr Badal Pal from Withington Hospital in Manchester agreed enthusiastically to review the material in this book and it's much the better for his input. He has also been one of the main supporting contributors to the NetDoctor website since it opened nearly three years ago and so it is a pleasure to acknowledge his invaluable help.

The Hodder & Stoughton editorial staff again deserve my sincere thanks for their help in producing another title in this series – you know who you are.

Great care is taken to ensure that the information presented here is accurate and if any error still exists then the responsibility is mine. Please let me know if you spot any mistakes or have any suggestions for improving these books. I can be contacted at d.rutherford@netdoctor. co.uk

Dr Dan Rutherford
Medical Director
www.netdoctor.co.uk

Chapter 1

What Is Arthritis?

Definitions

Arthritis is a general term that covers many medical conditions affecting the joints. A dictionary entry will generally run something like this:

Arthritis: *inflammation of one or more joints, accompanied by pain, stiffness, local heat, restriction of movement and redness of the overlying skin.*

Although these are all accurate enough features that may apply to an arthritic joint, such simple definitions belie the variety of forms that arthritis can take. For example the commonest of all types of arthritis affects the knees and the usual symptoms include pain and stiffness. However, an affected knee will not usually be noticeably hot, it often will not be swollen and the overlying skin will usually be a normal colour. Similarly someone might have quite severe arthritis of the spine, causing a lot of pain and stiffness yet just looking at the back can show nothing untoward.

A thumb just struck by a hammer during a spot of DIY will be sore, hot, swollen, stiff and red yet would not be considered to be arthritic because it will usually heal up completely in due course. Arthritis in a joint therefore implies a degree of permanence in the inflammation. Even if the symptoms wax and wane the implication of the term arthritis is that, even when the joint is quiet, a sufficiently detailed inspection of the inside of the joint would show that it is still inflamed to some extent.

Arthritis is an ominous word to most people when they first hear from a doctor that they have it in one or more joints. There is a common fear that arthritis will always get worse and that once it is present in one joint it is only a matter of time before it spreads through the rest of the body. Disability will then just be round the corner.

Such fears are usually misplaced. Arthritis is one of the commonest of all human conditions and the vast majority of people can live with it very well. Progress in the various treatments available has been steady over the past thirty or so years and many of the more dramatic developments, such as joint surgery, are now quite routine.

There are hundreds of medical conditions that can potentially be associated with joint disease. Rheumatology, as it is known, is one of the biggest specialities in medicine in terms of its scope. Much of the need in arthritis is therefore to cut through the complexities and to understand the basic principles of joints and how they work, what happens when they become arthritic and what can be done about this.

Synovial joints

Engineers and carpenters are familiar with a wide range of joints suited to different functions and the same is true of their equivalents in nature. Sometimes a joint is a junction between two parts of the bony structure of the body that are meant to be tightly held together and not to move much. An example is where each rib meets the breastbone. What we think of most though when referring to joints is a hinge that allows a large range of movement between two connected parts of the body. These are collectively known as the synovial (pronounced: *sigh-no-vee-al*) joints and it is worth knowing some details of their structure.

Synovial joints contain many highly specialised tissue cells and biological materials all custom designed to allow their internal surfaces to glide smoothly over each other through a wide range of movement, to bear loads of various degrees and yet remain stable and to function for a lifetime – when they are working properly. Large synovial joints such as the knee and hip have the same basic structure as small joints such as those of the fingers. This is shown in figure 1.

Essentially each synovial joint consists of two bone ends covered with a tough but smooth material called cartilage. This assembly is contained within a capsule composed of tough fibrous tissues attached

Figure 1: Normal synovial joint – a cross-section

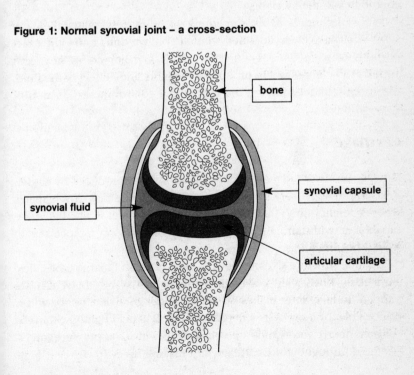

around each bone, near to the joint. The synovial capsule is a sealed 'bag' but has enough slack to allow the joint to move. The lining of this capsule is the synovium, which is a thin layer of special cells that produce a liquid called synovial fluid. This fluid not only lubricates the joint but it also nourishes the cartilage cells, because cartilage itself has no blood supply.

Only small amounts of synovial fluid are normally produced in a healthy joint – just enough to provide sufficient lubrication and to take oxygen and nutrients across the surface of the cartilage. Normal synovial fluid is clear and glue-like in its consistency whereas the fluid taken from an inflamed joint is runnier, due to the effect of the enzymes released by the inflamed joint. When an arthritic joint swells this is usually because of excess production of synovial fluid, which fills out the synovial capsule but thickening of the synovial tissues also contributes to the swelling.

Synovial fluid remains something of a mystery material. Many substances have been identified within it, but we don't know the exact purpose of each one. Hyaluronic acid is a major component and appears to be important in producing the lubricating effect of the fluid. Also poorly understood are the factors that control the production of synovial fluid.

Cartilage

Cartilage is one of the most remarkable substances produced by nature. It has to provide a very smooth, low-friction surface that closely mates with its neighbour so that the joint moves easily but it also has to be capable of withstanding a large amount of pressure, especially in weight-bearing joints.

The fine structure of cartilage is made of a mesh of large molecules, particularly one called collagen, within which water molecules are trapped. In fact water makes up about 70 per cent of cartilage and is responsible for most of its strength because it is held tightly within the collagen matrix and liquids are very able to withstand pressure forces. Scattered throughout the cartilage and making up 5–10 per cent of its volume are special cells, called chondrocytes (*kondro-sites*), which are responsible for the manufacture of collagen and the other materials that make up cartilage. The proper function of these cells is particularly important for maintaining healthy cartilage.

COLLAGENS

Actually there are 14 types of collagen in cartilage! All are constructed from three strands of protein wrapped around each other in a spiral (helix) shape. This arrangement gives collagen its great strength and the subtle differences between all the collagens gives them a range of other properties, such as flexibility.

Cartilage has different layers, each with slightly different properties suited to the precise role of that particular part of the joint. At the superficial level, where the cartilage is in contact with the synovial fluid and the cartilage from the other side of the joint there is relatively more collagen and less in the way of trapped water. This makes the superficial layer tougher and more resistant to wear and tear. Deeper within the cartilage there is less collagen and more water-trapping molecules so this region is more able to absorb shock loads and to cushion the effect of impact.

Cartilage is a living tissue and in common with all other parts of the body it is in a constant state of breakdown and repair. The chondrocytes are continually making new cartilage but also there are numerous enzymes active in breaking down old collagen and the other components for recycling. In a healthy joint these two processes are exactly balanced but in arthritis the breakdown process occurs more quickly than the repair.

This process of breakdown and renewal also occurs in the bone tissue that underlies the joint. Thus bones that are subjected to heavy loads can adapt by increasing manufacture and reducing destruction of bone, which thickens them up in areas that have to carry more weight, for example. Sometimes this process goes wrong, most notably in osteoporosis (chapter 11) where destruction goes ahead of repair and one ends up with weak bones.

Main types of arthritis

Damage to the cartilage is the central feature of all forms of arthritis, and it can occur by two main routes:

1 DEGENERATION

This is what happens in osteoarthritis – the commonest form of arthritis. Often this is called 'wear and tear' arthritis and it's not a bad label although it is important also to realise that osteoarthritis (OA) is an active process and not the inevitable fate of heavily used joints. In OA the load-bearing cartilage loses much of its trapped water content, which reduces its strength. The cartilage layer becomes thinner and breaks down, and abnormal mechanical stress is therefore transmitted through to the underlying bone. This causes the bone tissue to respond by thickening up in the region of the joint and also producing little spurs of bone (called osteophytes) at the edges of the joint. More details on osteoarthritis are in chapter 5.

2 INFLAMMATION

Inflammation means the body's response to any form of injury. A joint can therefore be inflamed due to trauma (the bashed thumb mentioned a few paragraphs ago) or infection (for example bacteria that have got into the bloodstream from another site in the body such as an infected wound and then settled within a joint). In these examples inflammation is the normal activity of the body's repair systems: removing dead tissue and bacteria for example. At the same time the repair part of the inflammatory process will also be active laying down new tissue to replace the damaged. Here, therefore, the inflammatory process is working as it should, in a positive way.

There is another type of tissue inflammation that is neither helpful nor necessary and which is responsible for inflammatory arthritis – the other main type. In this type of arthritis the immune system of the body attacks the synovial lining of the joints. In effect the body's immune system has turned against itself and this is therefore called an 'auto-immune' disease. There are many other types of auto-immune disease, each of which is usually specific to the type of tissue or organ that is being attacked. For example, Type 1 diabetes (insulin-dependent diabetes) is an auto-immune disease of the pancreas gland that results in the eventual failure of the pancreas to produce its own insulin.

The commonest inflammatory arthritis is rheumatoid arthritis (RA) and the inflammation of the synovium that occurs in RA results in the immune system also attacking the cartilage of the joint, and the adjacent bones. As synovial tissues are also part of the make-up of the tendons that attach muscles to bones these also become inflamed in RA. More details on RA and the effects it can have on tissues other than the joints are covered in chapter 7.

Key Points

- Arthritis means persistent inflammation of a joint.
- Synovial joints are those that are lined by cartilage, enclosed by a synovial capsule and designed to allow a large range of movement between the adjacent bones.
- The two main types of arthritis are degenerative (osteoarthritis) and inflammatory (rheumatoid arthritis).
- The inflammation in rheumatoid arthritis is an example of an auto-immune disease.

Chapter 2

The Causes of Arthritis

As with virtually every medical condition, our understanding of what causes the various forms of arthritis is patchy. Also in common with other diseases, it seems clear that it is the combination of many factors that is important and not the presence or absence of one particular causative agent. Often this is put as 'nature and nurture', meaning that someone might inherit a certain genetic tendency towards arthritis in their genes but whether they do or do not develop the condition then depends on factors within their environment and circumstances as they go through life.

HLA genes

Work on which genes might give rise to the tendency to certain types of arthritis is still in progress but some details have been well recognised for years. In particular is the association between what are known as the HLA (Human Leucocyte Antigen) genes and rheumatoid arthritis and also another form of arthritis called ankylosing spondylitis (chapter 8).

On the surfaces of most of our cells there are six proteins called 'HLA antigens'. Each cell in any one individual has the same six antigens but as there are about 150 HLA antigens known the exact combination of any six is unique to each human being (except identical twins, who share the same HLA type). When we hear of the need to find a matching tissue-type donor for an organ or bone marrow transplant it is the HLA type that people mean. Our HLA type is determined by our HLA genes, which are referred to by a letter/number code system. HLA-DRB1 is more common in white people with rheumatoid arthritis and over 95 per cent of whites with ankylosing spondylitis have the HLA-B27 gene.

Although the HLA genes are the most consistent yet shown to be associated with RA it is important to point out that RA is associated with a wide range of different types of gene patterns. Overall it is estimated that only about 30 per cent of someone's likelihood of developing RA will come from their genetic background.

Osteoarthritis and genes

There are several bits of circumstantial evidence that show the genes are also important in osteoarthritis (OA). For example there is a common type of OA that is seen in women around the time of the menopause that tends to distort the small joints of the fingers – they develop swellings at each of these joints, which then look knobbly. Often this type of arthritis later spreads to the knees and hips. The sister of a woman with this arthritis is three times more likely to develop it than the average woman.

Having a first degree relative (parent or sibling) with OA of the hand, knee or hip doubles a person's chance of also being affected.

These genetic 'clues' throw up as many questions as they do answers. For example 20 per cent of people with any form of OA have a positive family history of it. That also means that 80 per cent of people do not!

Risk factors

Having a family history of arthritis is therefore important but not a particularly good predictor of whether someone will develop the condition. It is a 'risk factor' and there are others known to be relevant to arthritis. The more risk factors someone has the more likely will they be to get arthritis. The main risk factors are:

AGE

Osteoarthritis is uncommon in people under 45 but if one takes X-rays of the joints of a group of people aged 65 then there is evidence of OA in at least half of them. One has to be cautious about drawing conclusions from this evidence, though, because X-ray appearances do not always tie up nicely with symptoms. You can have quite bad X-ray evidence of arthritis in a joint that gives few symptoms, and vice versa. Nonetheless the likelihood of having OA definitely increases as you get older. This might be due to the effect of increasing years of joint use, or a drop in the efficiency of the repair process within joints as we get older. Probably it is the combination of both.

Age is not a risk factor in RA – it occurs in all age groups although some increase is seen in women in their 20s and 30s.

SEX

Above age 55 OA is much more common in women, whereas in young people (under 45) men are more likely to be affected.

In younger people with RA women are more likely than men to be affected but in the older age groups the sexes are about even.

RACE

OA of the hip is less common in people of black, Asian or Chinese origin compared to whites. OA of the knee, however, affects these races more commonly, possibly due to habitual kneeling or sitting with the legs folded.

OBESITY

It would be logical to expect that OA of the load-bearing joints would be commoner in obese people and to some extent this is true. The association is strongest at the knee and in women. Very overweight women are several times more likely to develop knee arthritis than those who are lighter. Whether being overweight brings on the arthritis in the first place is debatable but the rate of deterioration of a joint affected by OA is certainly increased if the person is too heavy. Losing weight can significantly slow the pace of OA and is one of the most important things a person with OA can do to help themselves.

RA is not affected by weight but OA and RA can co-exist in the same person. In addition there are of course many other benefits to be gained from the avoidance of obesity, such as improved blood pressure, reduced cholesterol, reduced likelihood of developing diabetes and improved self-esteem.

HORMONES

Women with RA who become pregnant have often been observed to show an improvement in their arthritis during the pregnancy, which is presumably caused by their different hormone levels at that time. The oral contraceptive pill has at times been thought to protect against the development of RA but whether this is so is in some doubt. Possibly the pill can postpone the onset of RA. The gender differences seen in OA are presumably partly the result of hormonal differences between men and women but the contraceptive pill has no impact on OA.

PHYSICAL FACTORS

Trauma to a joint may predispose it to the development of OA later in life and occupations that involve a lot of kneeling and lifting of heavy weights have long been known to increase the risk of developing OA of the knees.

Professional sports people such as footballers and long-distance runners are at risk from both the increased loads on the knee and the greater chance of injury. Within the knee there are two extra cushioning pads of cartilage between the main joint surfaces that are prone to damage, particularly in footballers. These pads, called the menisci, need sometimes to be removed in an operation called meniscectomy if they are too badly worn. However, this markedly increases the likelihood of developing OA in that knee joint.

Uncommon contributory physical factors to the development of OA include childhood diseases such as Perthes' disease. This is a condition that affects the cap of the ball part of the ball and socket of the hip joint, i.e. the top of the femur or upper leg bone. This part, called the epiphysis, is an active area of growth and in Perthes' disease the cap slips into the wrong position, distorting the shape of the joint which then fails to form properly. Affected children are usually in the 4–8-year-old range but it can occur in children any age between 2 and 15. They will usually be noted to have a limp. Prompt treatment reduces the likelihood of long-term development of OA in the hip.

Congenital dislocation of the hip (CDH) is, as the name suggests, when a baby is born with the hips either dislocated or very prone to do so. For decades it has been part of routine baby checks in the UK to check for the presence of CDH and very few children now slip through the net. If treated early enough the results are excellent but there are many adults now with OA of the hip as a result of their CDH having been missed in an earlier era.

OTHER RISK FACTORS

Associations have been noted between OA, diabetes and high blood pressure but the reasons for these links are unknown. In the conditions called gout and pseudogout (chapter 10) osteoarthritis is associated with the appearance of crystals within the affected joint (of uric acid and calcium pyrophosphate respectively). In these conditions the crystals are deposited in the cartilage within the joints and may therefore cause local damage and lead to OA. At times, when these crystals are shed outside of the cartilage and into the joint space, they also cause acute pain and swelling in the affected joints such as the knees.

Haemochromatosis is a rare inherited condition in which too much iron is absorbed and stored in the body. Among the effects this can cause is OA, usually at an earlier age than is usual for OA.

These more uncommon types of OA related to other conditions are also peculiar in the joints they tend to affect, such as the second and third main knuckles in the hands (MCP joints). Usually it is rheumatoid rather than osteoarthritis that attacks these joints.

Protective factors

Osteoporosis (chapter 11) is the condition in which bone strength is below normal and surprisingly it has an opposite relationship to OA. Elderly people with osteoporosis are *less* likely to also have OA of the hip. Those with OA of the hip are generally found to have increased bone strength.

The relationship of smoking to arthritis is controversial. Some studies have suggested smokers are less commonly affected by OA. Bearing in mind that cigarette smoke contains around 8000 different chemical substances it is not difficult to imagine that, somewhere among the ammonia, arsenic, cyanide, lead, mercury, nicotine and all the other unpleasant materials inhaled every time someone lights up a cigarette, one of them might have an anti-inflammatory effect upon the joints. What is certain is that the risks of smoking outweigh any possible protection against arthritis that it might convey.

Key Points

- The causes of all forms of arthritis are a combination of genetic and environmental influences.
- There are very few definite gene links known in arthritis. The HLA genes recognised in many people with RA are the best recognised but their presence or absence does not predict whether someone will or will not get RA.
- OA is more common with increasing age.
- Most forms of arthritis are more common in women.
- Obesity and some occupations are strongly associated with the development of OA of the knees.
- OA of the hip is less likely to be found in people who have osteoporosis.

Chapter 3

Symptoms of Arthritis

THE SYMPTOMS OF JOINT DISEASE

It was mentioned in the previous chapter that X-ray surveys can show evidence of OA in about half of the population at the age of 65. By the age of 75, 80 per cent of people will have these X-ray changes. But if a joint that shows such evidence of OA gives no pain, moves well and isn't stiff or giving any trouble then we would have no reason to go to the doctor about it. In arthritis, therefore, it is the symptoms that matter and medical attention is therefore focused on those people who are bothered by their arthritis and take themselves along to their doctor about it. This contrasts with many other important medical conditions, such as high blood pressure for example, where there are few or no symptoms in the early stages and where the doctor has to look for the condition in order to treat it, often in someone who feels perfectly well!

Pain

Pain is the main symptom of any form of arthritis and is by far the commonest reason for consultation. There are some generalisations that one can make about the types and sites of pain that are helpful at the diagnostic stage.

Degenerative arthritis tends to give pain that improves with rest but gets worse with activity, and the opposite is true of inflamed joints. The person with OA is therefore at her best first thing in the morning and gets worse as the day goes by whereas in RA it takes a while for the person to get going and then once up to speed the rest of the day is not so bad.

The knee is the commonest site of OA and the inside tends to wear first, which is also where the pain tends to be – just on the inside of the joint at the level of the lower half of the knee cap.

Hip pain can be felt in the groin but commonly is 'referred' to the knee area. This occurs as a result of the way the pain-sensing nerves are connected at the lower end of the spine and can cause some confusion at times because the knee is where it hurts but the problem actually arises from an arthritic hip. Careful examination by the doctor will differentiate between the two.

Referral of pain is very common when the arthritis arises from the spine. Running the length of the spine, through the channel formed by the bony wings that project from the back of each of the vertebrae, is the spinal cord, which is connected to the rest of the body by the nerve branches that come off at each level between the vertebrae.

These fine nerves pass in bunches through the spaces between the spinal bones and in a healthy spine there is enough room for this all to happen easily. When arthritis attacks the spine there can be several consequences, among which are narrowing of the spaces between each vertebra and also the growth of bone spikes (osteophytes) between the vertebrae, all of which can compress the nerves en route to and from the spinal cord.

When a nerve that goes, say, to the outer aspect of the ankle is compressed or irritated by this process in the spine then, as far as the brain is concerned, the problem is coming from the ankle. The real problem is at the spinal nerve 'root' but the pain is *referred* by the brain to the source of the nerve. This is a common finding in spinal arthritis particularly of the lower back (where the radiation is down the buttocks or legs) or of the neck (where the radiation is down the shoulders or arms).

Stiffness

All arthritic joints tend to stiffen when they are rested. The time it takes them to ease off depends a bit on how active is the joint disease – very arthritic joints obviously take longer. In inflammatory arthritis it generally takes some hours for stiffness to decrease, whereas in OA the joints ease off much more quickly – within half an hour.

Swelling

An arthritic joint can be swollen for three reasons:

1 Thickening of the synovial tissues (the lining of the joint) and the surrounding capsule around the joint.
2 Extra synovial fluid within the capsule.
3 Bony swellings and deformity of the joint.

Any combination of the reasons can be present.

Synovial thickening is felt as a build-up of the tissues around the joint and this is also likely to be tender and hot to the touch. It usually indicates an inflammatory arthritis. Fluid within the joint may be slight and difficult to detect or, particularly in the case of the knee, be enough to make the joint several times larger than normal. There are different techniques that a doctor can use to detect excess synovial fluid (the technical term for which is an 'effusion'). In the knee for example, with the patient lying on his back and relaxing the leg muscles one can briskly push straight down on the kneecap and if there is a large effusion the kneecap will be felt to tap on the bones of the knee joint

Figure 2: Normal and arthritic hip joints

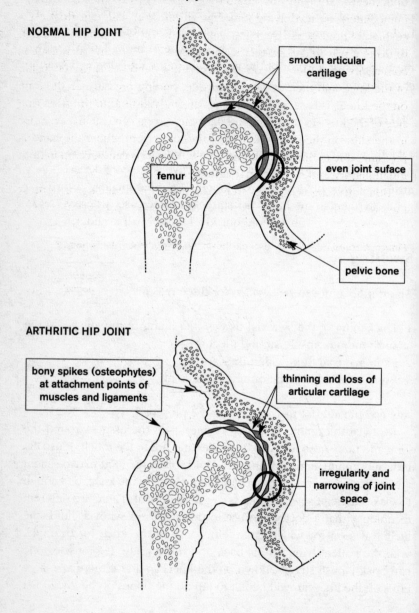

NORMAL HIP JOINT

smooth articular cartilage

even joint suface

femur

pelvic bone

ARTHRITIC HIP JOINT

bony spikes (osteophytes) at attachment points of muscles and ligaments

thinning and loss of articular cartilage

irregularity and narrowing of joint space

underneath. Normally this would not happen because the kneecap lies immediately on top of the joint but an effusion makes it float on a cushion of fluid. When there is a smaller effusion – perhaps not enough to make it possible to detect this 'tap' sign – then another technique is commonly used. Here the doctor sweeps his hand firmly up the inside of the knee and then down the outside, putting pressure all the time on the knee. This causes any excess of synovial fluid to flip from one side of the knee to the other and in doing so one can usually see a rise in the skin on the opposite side of the knee from where the hand is pressing, due to the fluid shifting across. Effusions can develop in both inflammatory and degenerative arthritis.

Bony swelling is typical of OA, due to the remodelling of bone at the sides of the joint and in particular the growth of osteophytes. Some

Figure 3: Hand affected by osteoarthritis, showing 'Heberden's nodes'

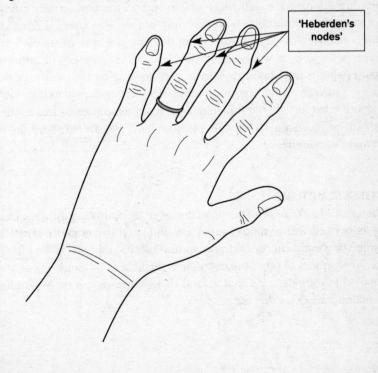

'Heberden's nodes'

of the main features of an arthritic (and the normal) hip are illustrated in figure 2. Despite the appearances such bony deformity does not always mean that the joint is either painful or restricted in function. A good example is the fingers of a woman with menopausal arthritis, which often runs in families (chapter 2). The nodules that develop at the end joints of the fingers are called Heberden's nodes (see figure 3) yet it is uncommon for someone to suffer much restriction of movement from fingers thus affected.

Problems caused by arthritis

The main importance of arthritis is the impact it has on mobility and the many aspects of daily living. A young and otherwise fit man might, for example, find that a minor degree of knee pain makes it very difficult for him to work as a roofer. An elderly person could find that their hip OA makes it difficult to get on and off the bus, so they rarely get into town. Arthritis can significantly impair someone's degree of independence – which is something that the majority of us wish to preserve as long as we possibly can. Less severe degrees of arthritis may just be a nuisance that flares up from time to time and can be easily controlled – the variations are endless. It is essential to take into account what exactly the difficulties are that the arthritis causes as this should be the main factor guiding how hard and by what means it should be treated.

OTHER SYMPTOMS

Rheumatoid arthritis, and the many forms of inflammatory arthritis, can be associated with symptoms that are unrelated to the joints, such as fatigue or weight change, skin rashes and other symptoms arising from the involvement of other organs such as the kidney or lungs. These are detailed in the relevant chapters and their presence can be important in making an exact diagnosis.

Chapter 4

Diagnosing Arthritis

When making any medical diagnosis a doctor combines the information from the patient's history with the results of clinical examination and laboratory tests. Tests are also very useful in monitoring the course of a condition – particularly the inflammatory types of arthritis such as RA – and to allow checks on the actions and side effects of the drugs used in treatment. A wide range of tests, including those on the blood, X-rays and tissue samples (such as of synovial fluid) can be applied in arthritis, although often very few are needed in any individual.

Within the time constraints of a busy general practice every GP has to use a form of shorthand assessment that reveals the necessary information in a short time. By far the commonest type of arthritis is osteoarthritis, so a focus on the particular joint in trouble along with a limited range of other tests or examinations is all that is necessary in the majority of patients. Experienced doctors become very good at recognising the patterns of common illnesses, so quite often a doctor will be able to make a confident diagnosis of OA based on the patient's history and a simple examination and with few if any other tests. When the diagnosis appears to indicate an inflammatory arthritis, or there is some variation from the routine types of OA ordinarily seen, or sometimes just to be sure that all other possibilities are eliminated, then other tests are done, as described below.

The majority of joint pains are seen and dealt with by GPs in the UK. Two types of specialists are commonly involved when the diagnosis is in doubt or the management of the arthritis needs more than can be offered by the GP alone – the rheumatologist and the orthopaedic specialist. Rheumatologists are physicians with special training in all aspects of arthritis and rheumatic diseases, whereas orthopaedic specialists are surgeons. Although most of the joint disease dealt with by orthopaedic surgeons is OA it is common for the two specialties to co-operate, particularly in the management of people with inflammatory joint disease such as rheumatoid arthritis.

Clinical assessment

By this is meant the examination carried out by a doctor (or other relevant health professional such as a physiotherapist), following on from listening to the patient's history. We covered one aspect – the detection of an effusion in the knee – in the previous chapter.

As doctors often refer to the various joints by their medical names, or the shorthand versions of them, it can be useful to know what they are before we go further:

Hands:
Knuckle joint = metacarpal-phalangeal (MCP)
Finger joint = interphalangeal (nearest to knuckle is the proximal interphalangeal 'PIP' and the furthest is the distal interphalangeal 'DIP')

Feet:
Base of toes (equivalent of knuckle in the hand) = metatarsal-phalangeal (MTP)

Fingers and toes are numbered from the thumb or big toe as the first, so a medical record that said '4th DIP' means the second finger joint on the ring finger and the 'first MTP' joint is the one at the base of the big toe.

A comprehensive but quick screen of all the joints that is used by many doctors is the 'GALS' screen – **G**ait, **A**rms, **L**egs and **S**pine. The main points are described here – so if you are subjected to it, you will realise what it's for!

GAIT
On walking one normally swings the arms and legs equally but pain of a shoulder or hip or knee joint will restrict its movement or cause a limp.

ARMS (INCLUDING HANDS)
The hands often give clues to help in making a more specific diagnosis in rheumatic conditions. Heberden's nodes, the bony knobbly swellings at the tips of the fingers (figure 3), are very likely to indicate OA. Such changes are likely to be in both hands with one or two fingers perhaps more affected than the others. In contrast, if there is thickening of the knuckles (MCP) and/or the middle small (PIP) joints of the fingers, then this is more likely to be due to RA especially if these changes are seen equally on both hands, and if the wrists are also affected (which are 'spared' in OA). In 'psoriatic' arthritis (chapter 8) various combinations of joint swellings are seen, often equally affecting both hands and wrists as in RA. Often, however, the pattern of joint involvement is asymmetric, i.e. on one hand say a knuckle joint is thickened while on the other hand perhaps just the wrist is affected and so on. Also, in

'psoriatic' arthritis, other patterns of involvement are seen, e.g. just one or two fingertip (DIP) joints are affected and nothing else.

If just one DIP finger joint suddenly swells and becomes red and painful then gout (chapter 10) is the likely diagnosis. Hence observing carefully the number and pattern of affected joints allows the doctor to make a fair guess at the likely diagnosis.

There are other well-recognised patterns that some types of arthritis take. For example, in longstanding RA the fingers swing away from the thumb and RA often limits a person's ability to touch the thumb to the index finger. It also can affect the elbow joint, making it more difficult to twist the forearms from the palm down to the palm up position.

Grip strength is assessed by squeezing the doctor's fingers. The shoulders are assessed by putting your hands behind your head and then bringing back the elbows.

LEGS

This is done with the person lying on his or her back on the examination couch. OA of the hip tends to make the leg draw up at the front and across to the other side. By moving the hip and then the knee it is possible to judge the degree of stiffness and restriction present at each. This is important in distinguishing between OA of the hip in which the pain is referred to the knee, and OA of the knee itself. One can also assess whether any of the toe joints are tender to squeezing – OA and gout commonly affect the main joint at the base of the big toe.

A useful test when assessing someone with low back pain that radiates down the legs is the 'straight leg raising test'. This detects limitation in the movement of the sciatic nerve – the main nerve that comes down the back of the leg and sends branches all the way to the toes. Normally the sciatic nerve has a degree of slack in its movement which allows it to slide up and down and so accommodate the curve it has to take around the buttocks when someone draws their leg up towards their tummy. If the nerves in the lower spine have become trapped by a bulge in the spongy discs between the vertebrae (a 'slipped disc') then the sciatic nerve is unable to slide back and forth so freely. To do the test the doctor asks the patient to keep the knee straight (which also stretches the sciatic nerve) and then he raises the patient's leg steadily, bending it at the hip. The point at which pain starts to appear in the back or down the leg signifies when the sciatic nerve has reached the end of its free movement and this is a rough measure of how big is the disc bulge. This test can be used to assess the progress of the disc problem – as it improves then the leg can be raised higher until eventually it should be possible to get the leg pointing straight up from the examination couch. More details on back pain and its treatment are in chapter 12.

Examining for the presence of an effusion in the knee has already been described but another finding that can be present if there is a lot of extra synovial fluid here is a so-called 'Baker's cyst'. This is not an occupational hazard of bread makers – Baker was a nineteenth-century surgeon who described the bulge at the back of the knee that now bears his name. It is due to excess synovial fluid going through to the back of the synovial capsule and causing a spongy swelling to appear. Occasionally a Baker's cyst can rupture, in which case the synovial fluid tracks downwards into the calf muscle. This can give rise to a situation that looks very like a clot in the leg veins (deep vein thrombosis) but tests done in hospital show which of the two it is.

SPINE

Looking carefully at the spine from the back will detect whether the line of the bones is straight: side-to-side curvature of the spine is called scoliosis. Scoliosis is not always obvious when looking at someone because people will unconsciously tilt their pelvis, raising one hip, to compensate if a scoliosis is pushing them off the vertical on standing. Getting the patient to lean forward is a technique that can make a scoliosis more noticeable because this causes the spine, and therefore the rib cage, to swing round so the ribs on one side of the back are then seen to be higher than the other side. There are many types of scoliosis and small degrees need not cause trouble. A form of severe scoliosis seen usually in adolescent girls is rare but important to detect and can require surgery to put right.

Forward curvature of the spine (seen from the side) is called kyphosis and to some extent this is a normal part of ageing. More obvious kyphosis is particularly seen in osteoporosis (chapter 11), when the weakness of the vertebrae causes them to crumple at their front edges. A little bit of crumpling at several vertebrae can result in quite a noticeable kyphosis.

By asking the patient to bend forward and try touching his or her toes the doctor assesses the flexibility of the lower spine. However, one needs to check that movement is actually occurring between the vertebrae (usually done by placing two fingers in the gaps between adjacent vertebrae). This is to eliminate the false impression one might get from someone who has flexible hips yet a stiff spine (for example due to ankylosing spondylitis – chapter 8)

Human beings turn their heads a lot from side to side, so the degree of wear between the vertebrae in the neck is high and over the years this often causes OA of the spine here. An early sign of this is reduced movement of the neck from side to side, which is tested by trying to touch the ear to the shoulder while keeping the shoulders level.

Blood tests

Although blood tests can be very helpful in making a precise diagnosis in inflammatory arthritis they generally show little or nothing abnormal in degenerative arthritis. They cannot predict if someone will or won't get any sort of arthritis in the future and they often do not add much or anything to the accuracy of the diagnosis reached just by listening to the history and doing a skilful clinical examination. Much of the time a doctor will check the 'bloods' in someone with joint pains to double check if anything else might be happening, for example in other body systems such as the liver, kidneys or thyroid gland. More often than not it is used as a reassurance for the patient who otherwise seems pretty clearly to have a straightforward diagnosis of osteoarthritis. It is therefore important to get the value of blood tests in perspective.

Because in inflammatory arthritis the immune system is intimately involved in the disease process a very large number of tests are now available that can potentially help define the exact type of arthritis, and the degree of activity of the inflammation. This is of particular value in deciding upon and monitoring the effect of treatment – both in terms of its effectiveness and also in looking out for the possible side effects of the drugs used. Particularly in RA many of the drugs need careful monitoring to ensure that side effects are kept to a minimum. These are dealt with in chapter 7.

The details of most of the tests available to rheumatologists are best left for them to know and interpret! There are, however, a smaller number of tests used more often than the rest that are useful to know something about:

ERYTHROCYTE SEDIMENTATION RATE (ESR)

Plasma is the straw-coloured liquid component of blood – the other main component being the red cells that carry oxygen. About half of blood is plasma and the other half red cells and of course in life the two components are completely mixed. If one takes a blood sample and places it in a tall glass tube, adds material to prevent the blood from clotting and then just leaves it alone, over a period of a few hours the red cells will slowly settle to the bottom half of the tube. The rate at which the red cells fall has long been known to be a crude measure of the degree of activity of the immune system of the person from whom the blood sample has been taken. As the proper medical name for red blood cells is 'erythrocytes' the rather grand name for this simple test is the 'erythrocyte sedimentation rate', universally abbreviated to 'ESR'. For decades the ESR has been the common test used by doctors the world over to measure 'inflammation'. To be exact it is the number of millimetres fallen in an hour by a column of red blood cells, when measured under certain standard conditions. The greater the inflammation (from whatever cause, be it arthritis, infection or a host of other possibilities) then the greater is the ESR. Normal blood has a value of about 20mm or less.

What alters the rate at which red cells settle is largely the composition of the protein molecules within the plasma, and many of these proteins are made by the immune system. Hence with increased inflammation there are more such proteins, which make the red cells clump together and these clumps (still microscopically small) fall more quickly than the individual red cells would. The same physics determines that large hailstones fall faster than flakes of snow.

The ESR has fallen out of popularity in recent years for various reasons. For example, it can be inaccurate if someone is anaemic (in which case they have fewer red cells to start with) and it is elevated by a host of factors that have nothing to do with inflammation, such as gender, cholesterol, age, obesity and pregnancy. The original technique involved blood lying in tubes, which in these days of increased awareness of biological hazard is no longer an acceptable practice. Better test kits are now available though and as the test is easy, quick and cheap to do it will probably remain useful for many years yet, despite its limitations.

PLASMA VISCOSITY (PV)

The ESR is an indirect measure of the 'thickness' or viscosity of the plasma, as determined by its protein content, so the more sophisticated successor to the ESR has been to measure the viscosity of the plasma directly. Plasma viscosity is more accurate, does not vary between the sexes and is independent of other factors such as anaemia.

C-REACTIVE PROTEIN (CRP)

This is a protein produced by the immune system when there is inflammation going on somewhere in the body. Many doctors find it more useful than the ESR as it is more immediately sensitive to changes in the level of inflammation.

Exactly which test is used where and when varies a lot from doctor to doctor and between the different regions in the UK. Some hospital laboratories have their own preferences. Each test has its pros and cons and there isn't any clear best test.

ANTIBODIES

Antibodies are proteins produced by the immune system in response to an attack of some sort. As we've seen, in inflammatory arthritis the immune system attacks the synovial tissues of the joints, and a number of antibodies can be found in conditions like RA that take part in this auto-immune process. Of the many possible antibody tests used by rheumatology specialists three are the most common:

- **Rheumatoid factor**: as the name suggests this is most commonly found in the blood of people with RA, and high levels of rheumatoid factor can indicate that someone's RA is particularly active. However, up to nearly a third of people with RA are negative for rheumatoid factor in the blood and 15 per cent of healthy people over 65, with no evidence of RA, are positive for rheumatoid factor.
- **Anti-nuclear antibodies**: useful markers of inflammation but are present in about 8 per cent of people without arthritis.
- **Anti-DNA antibody**: the presence of anti-DNA antibody is highly suggestive of a condition called systemic lupus erythematosus (SLE – see chapter 9). Anti-nuclear antibodies are also often found in SLE.

X-rays

It's generally true to say that X-rays are over-used by doctors in dealing with arthritis. They rarely provide information that changes a diagnosis made on clinical grounds and often add nothing to the management of someone's arthritis. Doctors, particularly GPs, often find themselves under pressure to request an X-ray simply because the patient expects it to be done. It can happen that one very occasionally sees something unexpected on an X-ray but for the majority of people with joint pains in the knees, hips and back the X-ray is not much help. Although modern equipment uses very low doses of radiation exposure it is best to avoid it whenever possible. The financial and manpower costs to the health service of unnecessary X-rays are very large indeed.

The circumstances when an X-ray is helpful (or not) can be summarised thus:

- **Knees**: helpful when symptoms are so severe or troublesome that referral to an orthopaedic specialist has become necessary. The X-ray will help the surgeon decide on the appropriateness of surgery to the knee.
- **Hips**: as for knees, i.e. when an orthopaedic opinion is being sought.
- **Spine (back pain)**: when the pain has gone on for several weeks and is responding poorly to treatment.
- **Neck**: arthritis of the neck is common and can be confirmed by simple clinical examination so most of the time neck X-rays are of little or no additional value. An important exception is in someone with rheumatoid arthritis, which, rarely, can cause instability of the top two neck vertebrae that can be detected by X-rays with the neck in different positions.

In fact there always have to be exceptions – for example if there is something unusual on examination or the history is not typical for arthritis. Then it is perfectly reasonable to do an X-ray to confirm what is going on. Usually there will be a clue that points to the unexpected, and of particular importance is the history of trauma. Sudden onset hip or back pain in an elderly person who had a stumble a few days previously might turn out to be a fracture of the hip or spine for example.

The hands are perhaps a special case. We've previously mentioned 'menopausal' arthritis and this has several features that make it quite easily recognisable. However, the hands can be affected in different ways in several types of inflammatory arthritis and the diagnosis of which type it is can be helped by examining the details of the small hand joints on an X-ray. So if someone's blood tests came back with a raised ESR or PV or CRP and they also had pain in the hand joints then a hand X-ray could make the diagnosis more precise.

Synovial fluid

If there is enough fluid in an arthritic joint such as the knee to cause it to swell up then it is usually quite easy for a doctor to take a sample of the fluid using a syringe and fine needle. The likelihood of getting useful information from a synovial fluid sample goes up as the number of painful joints goes down. If someone therefore has a single hot swollen knee then a synovial fluid examination will be the best way to ensure that it is not an infected joint or gout, because these are both conditions that typically attack one joint at a time.

Infection of a joint is known as septic arthritis and in the UK it is now fortunately a rare problem. Nonetheless it is a potentially very serious one, not just for the joint (which can be rapidly and severely damaged by bacteria) but also because septic arthritis can be part of or give rise to blood poisoning, which even in our antibiotic age has a high mortality and needs prompt diagnosis and treatment. Septic arthritis should be suspected if a single joint rapidly becomes inflamed and there are other signs of infection such as a fever or chills. The synovial fluid would be likely to reveal the infecting bacteria and large numbers of inflammatory cells or pus.

More common than septic arthritis is gout, which is due to the settling out in the joint of crystals of a naturally occurring substance called uric acid. Under the microscope uric acid crystals have a characteristic needle shape. Detecting uric acid crystals in the synovial fluid from an inflamed joint makes the diagnosis of gout certain.

If there are several inflamed joints it is much more likely that the person has an inflammatory or degenerative arthritis, in which case the synovial fluid will probably not add much to what is already known or suspected. However, it can be difficult to be certain of the nature of a particular person's arthritis despite all the other tests we've mentioned, and then the findings from synovial fluid analysis might be the only way to make the correct diagnosis. Even so, the fluid from even a very inflamed joint may only reveal some non-specific abnormalities. As with most medical tests, synovial fluid analysis is not infallible.

Diagnosis in practice

Medical textbooks deal with individual diseases and their accompanying features and test results in nice neat chapters. To make it easier there are even separate books for rheumatology and skin disease and heart disease and so on down the list of specialties. The first time a student doctor meets a live patient he or she discovers that in real life people do not walk out of textbooks with a clear list of symptoms and signs. Instead it can look as though someone has taken all the pages out of all of the books and shuffled the lot together.

One of the commonest reasons for people to go to their doctor is because of joint pain. Sometimes, however, the symptoms of arthritis are not so straightforward. Rather than pain some people notice tingling or numbness, or complain of 'circulation' problems or 'muscle aching' or 'stiffness' or even just not feeling well or simply 'tired'. Sometimes it will be easy for the doctor to say right away what is wrong, but more often it will be difficult to be sure. As we've seen from the earlier sections of this chapter, all the available tests have their limitations, and deciding what is the cause of joint pain often comes down to pattern recognition – knowing what sort of symptoms make one diagnosis more likely than another and then applying tests and putting those results into the mix as well.

If the 'inflammation' tests are normal (ESR, PV, CRP), antibody tests are negative and there are no other symptoms to suggest a more generalised sort of illness then it will be very likely that OA (or some other non-inflammatory condition) is the cause. If the person has felt generally tired or perhaps lost weight and if the inflammation tests are positive then an inflammatory condition like RA is more likely. If a single joint (particularly the base of the big toe) is very painful, with swelling and redness, then it is gout that is most likely.

Sometimes it remains unclear what the exact diagnosis is. For example, someone might have joint pains but they don't follow a consistent pattern, or the joints look perfectly normal on examination and all the tests are negative (including in inflammatory arthritis). It might then be best just to wait and see how the pains develop over the next few months, provided they are not causing too much trouble. Some virus illnesses for example can cause temporary joint pains that go away after some weeks or months. It can be particularly hard to be certain what has caused back pain and how long it will last.

If simple painkiller drugs dampen the symptoms and there are no special features on examination and testing then there is really no hurry to make a more precise diagnosis. If the symptoms cannot be controlled easily, or the side effects of treatment are too much, or there are other features that don't quite add up then it can be necessary for a rheumatologist to see the person and make the diagnosis.

Key Points

- Diagnosing the cause of joint pains is often not an exact or definite process.
- The points that help most to make a diagnosis are the history of the development of the pain and the findings on simple examination by the doctor.
- Blood tests have a limited value in diagnosing arthritis but are of most use in inflammatory types such as rheumatoid arthritis.
- X-rays are of little value in the diagnosis and management of the majority of people with joint pain.
- Extra tests such as sampling synovial fluid are most likely to be helpful when only one or a few joints are involved.

Chapter 5

Osteoarthritis

In people over the age of 65, osteoarthritis is by far the commonest disorder that affects joints. It is first and foremost a disease of the cartilage, which at first patchily and then progressively becomes weaker and then splits and breaks up. Looking at the surface of a severely arthritic joint it is easy to appreciate that it should also be painful and stiff but OA is a condition that is as mysterious as it is common, and there are many questions about it that remain unanswered.

Why, for example, should it be that about half of people who have X-ray evidence of fairly marked OA will have no complaints about the joint examined? Why is it that arthritic joints are painful when cartilage has no nerve fibres within it to detect pain? Despite being so common, OA is poorly understood. Perhaps unfortunately it lacks the glamour of heart surgery or the cutting edge interest of gene technology but it is responsible for a huge personal, social and economic burden of disease throughout the world.

The known factors that increase the risk of developing OA were covered in chapter 2. Obesity is the strongest risk factor, particularly for the knees and especially for younger people.

It is a common worry that having OA in one joint inevitably means that it will spread to the rest. Generally this is not the case, although it is true that OA can get steadily worse in any of the joints affected, usually over a period of years. As yet we do not have medicines that can significantly alter the rate at which OA progresses, or which can reverse the trend and promote healing of arthritic joints. This is an area where drug companies are heavily involved in research – a treatment that reverses or even slows the development of OA would be tremendously valuable, both to sufferers of OA and to the manufacturers of the drug.

Assessing osteoarthritis treatment

Because we lack medicines that tackle the disease itself the treatment of OA in practice means controlling its symptoms – pain, stiffness and restriction of movement. One of the difficulties in judging the value of treatments is that people vary considerably in the extent to which they will experience symptoms despite apparently similar levels of arthritis. Some people with little evidence of joint disease might complain of a lot of pain, whereas others with apparently more severe arthritis might be better at putting up with discomfort and therefore report fewer symptoms.

Studies on OA treatment effects have to rely heavily on 'subjective' measurements such as scores of the amount of pain experienced by the patient over a period of time. Such methods are prone to being less accurate and more difficult to do than tests for medical conditions that can be independently measured in some way. For example, high blood pressure is a very common problem that often requires drug treatment. One can use a machine to measure a person's blood pressure quite accurately so it is easy to prove whether a particular treatment to lower the pressure works, and to what degree. The blood pressure level can therefore be measured 'objectively' and free of any bias from the patient's ability to put up with it being raised.

Of all the possible factors capable of producing misleading information in assessing the effect of treatment one of the most powerful is the 'placebo effect'.

Placebo effect

Human beings may respond positively to any treatment if they have enough faith that it will work. One could, for example, manufacture pills with completely inactive materials but call them painkillers. If then given to people suffering pain with enough conviction that they were effective there would undoubtedly be a proportion of them who would be convinced their pains were relieved. This is the placebo effect, the effect one could say of mind over matter, and it is a force that has to be reckoned with in almost every field of medicine.

To make allowances for the placebo effect it is common in medical research studies to have at least two groups of patients with the medical condition that one is trying to treat, one half of whom are given the experimental treatment and the other half are given the placebo. The commonest treatments examined this way are new drugs, in which case the placebo pills would be made to look exactly the same as the 'real' drug. In the best studies these two treatment groups are swapped over half way through the investigation period and the details of which group has which treatment is kept secret from all of the patients and most of the researchers until the end of the study, when the codes are broken. All of the patients will therefore experience the placebo effect but they won't know when they were receiving active drug or placebo. If the drug being tested actually works then it will be clear that the results during treatment with it are substantially better than the placebo groups.

A symptom like pain is particularly vulnerable to the placebo effect, which is why such a range of arthritis treatments, including bizarre diets and impossible remedies such as metal wristbands, all have their devotees. As we'll see shortly, new research indicates that even some widely used conventional treatments such as surgical washing-out of arthritic knees might be no better than placebo. Therefore at least some of what until now we have considered to be the right way to treat arthritis may really have no true value – which is quite a hard concept for doctors and patients to accept.

Painkillers

Pain is the commonest symptom of OA, and mild to moderate pain responds quite well to simple painkillers (analgesics) in most people. Paracetamol tablets are the most commonly prescribed. Codeine, dihydrocodeine and dextropropopoxyphene are opiate-based pain-killers (see below) that are commonly mixed with paracetamol to give combinations that are 'stronger' than paracetamol alone. The names of the combinations thus formed are, respectively: co-codamol, co-dydramol, and co-proxamol. (Full details of all the drugs commonly used to treat arthritis are in appendix B.)

PARACETAMOL

Paracetamol has been proven to give better pain relief than placebo, but only in fairly short-term studies in people with arthritis (this time limitation applies to much of the medical research in joint disease). OA of course is basically a permanent condition, although it usually has its ups and downs, but many people therefore need to take analgesics for years. In overdose, or in someone who has significant liver disease, paracetamol is potentially toxic or even fatal. When used at no more than the full recommended dose by people who do not have any problems with their liver it is a safe drug, including in the long term. To get the most benefit from any analgesic it needs to be used at the correct dose. For paracetamol that is two tablets (1g) every six hours. Many people use painkillers too infrequently or at less than full dose, which is often why they don't get adequate pain relief.

CODEINE

The main side effects with codeine and drugs like it are nausea and constipation, which can limit the usefulness of combination drugs in many people. Addiction to codeine can also occur and some people undoubtedly do develop some dependence on their painkillers. If someone has severe pain though it can be almost impossible to separate their need for pain relief from the possibility that they are dependent on the painkiller – for both reasons they will need the next dose of the medicine. Provided one always uses the least powerful drug to control the symptoms then this is a problem that cannot be completely avoided. One has to live with the fact that no drug is perfect, and if a certain medication gives good relief of symptoms and so improves someone's quality of life, then it sometimes has to be accepted that some side effects have to be tolerated in order to achieve the desired result.

Soluble versions of the common paracetamol/codeine preparations do not work any better than the non-soluble ones at relieving pain. They are often more expensive than ordinary tablets and some of them contain quite a lot of salt (sodium) which is a potential problem for some people with heart or kidney complaints. They are best restricted to people who find it difficult to swallow solid tablets.

ASPIRIN

Aspirin is the other main simple painkiller. It is much less commonly used for pain relief now because of its tendency to cause stomach upset (ulcers and bleeding from the digestive system). Low dose aspirin is however very widely used in many of the medical conditions associated with the heart and blood vessels, as it reduces the tendency of the blood to clot. At these low doses it has little or no pain-killing effect.

OPIATE ANALGESICS

We could do with more choice in painkillers like paracetamol but so far medical research has not discovered them. All the other available analgesics are related in some way to morphine – the active compound derived from the opium poppy and the top of the pecking order of potency. The other collective medical name for this class of analgesics is therefore the 'opiate' or 'opioid' group.

There are about twenty opiates now available for prescription. Apart from the combinations of paracetamol with codeine-like drugs already mentioned, dihydrocodeine and tramadol account for most of the other opiates in common use for OA. They offer only modest, if any, improvement over simple analgesics in their pain-relieving power but tramadol is probably less likely to cause constipation and addiction, although occasionally it causes other unpleasant side effects such as confusion or even hallucination.

NON-STEROIDAL ANTI-INFLAMMATORY DRUGS (NSAIDS)

This group of drugs is now one of the most widely used throughout the world for a range of conditions, of which pain relief is the commonest. Ibuprofen is the 'typical' NSAID and the only one that can be bought in the UK without a prescription.

NSAIDs are effective but they are also associated with several important problems, with the result that about a quarter of all drug-related side effects reported in the UK are caused by this class of drug. There are many issues concerning their use and safety, some of which are the subject of current controversy in the medical community. So important are NSAIDs that they are given more detailed coverage in the next chapter. Only the information particularly relevant to OA is therefore presented here.

In brief, the use of NSAIDs for osteoarthritis used to be frowned upon by rheumatologists on the basis that OA was just a passive 'wearing-away' of joints and not due to tissue inflammation like rheumatoid arthritis. Patient experience showed, however, that many people with OA got good pain relief from NSAIDs, and subsequent medical research has also shown that OA is an active inflammatory process too, even if we don't understand it well. So there is sound logic in using NSAIDs for OA.

Ibuprofen remains the logical first-choice NSAID for the vast majority of people. It comes in several strengths of tablet and in liquid form as well as a gel that is effective when rubbed on the skin. It is also cheap and available without prescription. When purchasing ibuprofen there is no advantage in spending extra money on a 'branded' product with fancy packaging. Simple ibuprofen tablets in a plain box contain the same active ingredient. If someone pays for their prescriptions and needs ibuprofen long term it will usually be cheaper for them to get a couple of months' supply at a time from their GP rather than to go on buying them across the counter.

'Alternative' painkillers

There has always been a great deal of interest in alternative medicines for OA. Partly these are rooted in history – arthritis has been detected in the earliest of human remains and people have always sought remedies for it. In modern times alternative treatments have enjoyed a tremendous surge in popularity for many reasons. Partly some people wish to avoid what can be significant problems associated with modern drugs, whereas others favour 'natural' treatments on matters of principle.

In studying the effects of the many alternative treatments available modern medical science runs up against several problems that make the task difficult to do. First there is always the placebo effect to deal with – which can be particularly strong in some alternative treatments with their sometimes quite strong undertones of faith. Even when the treatment under scrutiny is a herb or other compound there can be significant problems in measuring the strength of the active ingredient. One batch of herbal treatment might therefore be considerably less or more active than another batch, so comparisons between different groups of patients or over long periods of time can be almost impossible.

These difficulties can make it very difficult even for open-minded 'conventional' doctors to recommend such treatments to their patients. Such well-founded caution can be misinterpreted by enthusiasts for complementary treatments as proof that orthodox medicine is always at loggerheads with their interests. Historically this might have been true, but modern medical science is now much more interested in bridging the gaps between these different methods of treatment. 'Complementary' as opposed to 'alternative' is therefore a more appropriate term to use and implies that the various disciplines can be used together, rather than in isolation from each other. This integrated approach to the variety of medical practice is already quite well developed in the USA and is beginning to gain momentum in Europe. As yet, however, only a handful of complementary treatments for arthritis have been subjected to the sort of investigation that is routine for prescription medicines. Two substances that have been looked at are glucosamine and chondroitin.

Glucosamine and chondroitin

Chondroitin is the main component of what is called the 'ground substance' of cartilage. This is the water-trapping material that fills in the mesh made by the collagen fibres and which, as we've seen, gives cartilage its strength under pressure and smooth surface. Chondroitin is manufactured by cells scattered throughout the cartilage.

Glucosamine is a complex molecule derived from glucose (sugar) and is one of the main starting points for the manufacture within the body of many other compounds, including hyaluronic acid (found in synovial fluid) and other components of cartilage.

Glucosamine and chondroitin are 'raw materials' used in the construction of cartilage, which is probably why taking supplements of them has come about as a treatment. Generally, however, the metabolism of the body is far more sophisticated than this concept suggests. For example, the protein of a beefsteak is very similar to the protein of a human muscle, but swallowing a piece of steak does not directly result in any growth of the diner's biceps! Instead the digestive system breaks down the complex proteins within steak into simpler components, which are absorbed and utilised in a number of processes, including the building of other proteins, which may or may not be muscle, within that person's body.

So the idea that taking in a supplement of glucosamine or chondroitin will result in either of these materials finding their way through the digestive system, bloodstream and then to the joint of an arthritic person where they will be laid down to reinforce the worn cartilage stretches the credulity of most scientists and medical professionals. Such information as exists, however, suggests that for once this scepticism may be unjustified – glucosamine and chondroitin have both been shown to relieve the pain of arthritis to a greater extent than can be accounted for by the placebo effect.

The best study published to date looked at people aged over 50 who had knee arthritis and who were given either glucosamine or placebo over a three-year period (see appendix A for references). The treated group had a significant improvement in their levels of pain and stiffness. The researchers also examined detailed X-rays of the knees of the people who took part in the study, looking in particular at the thickness of the cartilage within the joints. The people treated with glucosamine seemed to show a lower rate of loss of cartilage than the placebo group.

No exactly similar studies have yet been done for chondroitin but there is some evidence that it is effective in reducing arthritis symptoms. There is no research comparing chondroitin and glucosamine against each other. Many people take both and they appear to be free of any important side effects.

There are literally hundreds of advertisements in magazines and in particular on the internet for these preparations and certainly many of the claims for them are wildly exaggerated. Some arthritis experts feel that the evidence for glucosamine and chondroitin is very weak if present at all – they are certainly not cure-alls for arthritis. They do agree that it is safe and probably worth a try. This, however, begs the question of which one to use, and how much of it? There is no internationally agreed dosage or standardisation of these materials, such as is rigorously applied to standard prescription drugs. The three-year study referred to above used 1500 milligrams daily of glucosamine yet some commercial preparations available in the UK contain only 100 milligrams per capsule. It is possible for a GP to prescribe glucosamine and chondroitin on the NHS, but they are not officially listed medicines and so it is up to the individual doctor's discretion whether he or she will be willing to issue them. It is also possible to purchase them without a prescription, and the best advice for someone wishing to do so is to discuss the matter with a pharmacist. The cheapest preparation is likely to be as good as any other.

Herbal medicines

There are probably hundreds of plant remedies for arthritis around the world, and making scientific sense of what works, or at least might be worth a try, is a huge task. Fortunately several recent reviews have been made of this area and full details of the references are in appendix A. The following list is not exhaustive but presents some of the main herbal remedies that may be effective in osteoarthritis. Although there are few if any serious side effects known with the listed preparations it is wise to discuss using them with a pharmacist rather than without advice. In most of the studies done on these medicines the positive effects, when present, were small and most used only small numbers of patients over fairly short time scales, so the results might not be representative of their true value.

CAPSAICIN CREAM

Capsaicin is familiar to anyone who has ever eaten a curry as it is what makes chillies and peppers 'hot'. If you have ever chopped a chilli and then unwisely touched your face without washing your hands you will also know that capsaicin can be intensely irritating to the skin. Capsaicin cream applied several times a day can reduce the pain of arthritis, which it may do partially by acting as a 'counter-irritant'. This means essentially that the nerve fibres conducting pain signals from the arthritic joint are partially blocked by the activity in the skin nerves. Another theory is that capsaicin forces a drop in the local concentration of a substance within nerve fibres that is used in sending pain signals to the brain. It can take weeks for capsaicin to work but for some people the amount of pain relief is considerable. For others the cream irritates the skin too much or doesn't help. Capsaicin is prescribable on the NHS.

AVOCADO/SOYBEAN EXTRACTS

Oils from avocado and soybeans are mixed and from the combination an extract called avocado/soybean unsaponifiables (thankfully more commonly called 'ASU') has been used to some positive effect on OA of the hip and knee. It can take several months to work and only the oral (capsule) form has been analysed for effectiveness (ASU also comes in cream form).

WHITE WILLOW BARK

This is an old traditional remedy but one of the ingredients of white willow bark is salicin, which is an aspirin-like compound. Salicin is also present in some other herbal products.

DEVIL'S CLAW

This is a plant native to Africa, extracts of which are available in capsule form. In fairly short trials (up to two months) it appeared to give pain relief in OA.

CHINESE AND AYURVEDIC PREPARATIONS

Thunder God Vine is a Chinese remedy for rheumatoid arthritis for which there is some evidence of effectiveness. An Ayurvedic medicine called Articulin-F seems to be of some benefit in OA.

Other treatments

Treatments other than painkillers abound for arthritis. Chiropractic, therapeutic massage, reflexology, homeopathy, osteopathy and aromatherapy are just some of the many available and it is impossible in a book of this nature to give them more than a mention. This does not mean that they have no value – quite the reverse is true if the popularity of these treatments is any guide. Unfortunately few of them have been subjected to detailed medical study and it is therefore impossible to present them in the same context as 'conventional' treatments. No form of complementary treatment for arthritis has been consistently shown to provide better results than placebo in published trials but it would be unfair to therefore dismiss them as possible choices for someone with severe joint problems.

Acupuncture can help in pain relief as an extra option, as can transcutaneous electronic nerve stimulation (TENS). TENS delivers tiny electrical impulses from a portable battery-powered unit to small electrodes placed on the skin near the painful area. It probably works a bit like counter-irritation, by blocking the ability of nerve fibres to conduct pain signals. TENS machines can be bought but advice on their use is best sought from a health professional such as a physiotherapist. Many physiotherapy or rheumatology departments are able to lend a TENS machine to a patient for a while to see if it helps.

Often one of the most difficult issues for someone wishing to try complementary medicine is how to find a properly qualified practitioner. Contact addresses for some of the relevant organisations that control standards or hold lists of practitioners are in appendix C.

Physiotherapy

As well as causing pain, joint disease causes stiffness and impairs mobility. Physiotherapists are the healthcare professionals who are skilled in helping people regain lost function by a number of means including remedial exercise, massage, manipulation and other techniques. They have an important role to play in rehabilitating someone after joint surgery and in conjunction with colleagues from other disciplines, such as occupational therapy, in helping someone with more severe arthritis adapt their way of living to help them cope.

Much as we'd like them to have magical powers, in reality they can't cure arthritis either. Someone with arthritis will often be sent to a physiotherapist by their doctor after the diagnosis of OA is made, with sometimes unrealistically high expectations on both sides of what that will achieve. Physiotherapy is more about being shown how to help yourself if you have OA, than it is about having treatment 'done' to you. The people who benefit most from physiotherapy are those who put into practice the advice that the physiotherapist gives.

Some techniques that have been long used in physiotherapy appear to have no definite value, such as ultrasound treatment. Ultrasound is high frequency sound waves, which are used in a variety of medical applications, particularly in obtaining images from within the body – the familiar pregnancy scan uses ultrasound. Ultrasound has been thought to benefit healing in arthritis for years but a recent review showed no benefit from it in people with knee arthritis.

One small study of 14 patients showed that applying tape to push the kneecaps inwards (i.e. towards the opposite leg) reduced pain in people with knee arthritis. This probably works by shifting the load-bearing surfaces of the underside of the kneecap and adjacent knee joint slightly, relieving the pressure on the most arthritic parts. This study looked at the effect of taping for just a few days, so does not answer the question of how effective it might be over a long period of time. It is a harmless treatment that is worth trying, and a physiotherapist can teach someone how to apply the tape for themselves.

Joint fluid removal and injections

SYNOVIAL FLUID REMOVAL

Particularly within the knee joint, one of the responses of an arthritic joint is the excess production of synovial fluid. So much fluid can be produced that the knee visibly swells, usually in front but often also at the back, producing a Baker's cyst (chapter 4). This excess fluid may have some benefit in providing extra cushioning for the joint, but it also can lead to problems. All fluids resist compression, and during walking the knee joint is, of course, under pressure. The excess fluid can impair the range of movement of the joint and so one of the simplest, if temporary, ways of relieving the pain and stiffness of a severely arthritic joint is to remove some of the excess synovial fluid. This can be done using no more than a needle and a syringe and is an easy technique that can be performed by most GPs. Care has to be taken to avoid introducing infection into the joint but this is not difficult to ensure. Removing 10 or 20 millilitres of fluid can markedly lower the joint pressure and give an extra degree of freedom of movement. Unfortunately the improvement is usually quite short-lived if this is all that is done.

JOINT 'WASHOUT' (LAVAGE)

This is a procedure (also called 'tidal irrigation') undertaken sometimes by orthopaedic surgeons where a wide-bore hypodermic needle is inserted into a joint (e.g. the knee), through which sterile fluids are run in to the joint and let out by another needle inserted at the opposite side of the joint. It is undertaken in mild to moderately affected OA joints with the idea that harmful joint fluids and 'debris' can be washed out to produce some benefit including pain relief. This procedure has to be performed as an in-patient and under very clean conditions to avoid introducing infection.

Joint lavage is a commonly done procedure but its value has been severely questioned by a recent American study, which showed it was no better than 'dummy' treatment, i.e. placebo. It is far harder to run a placebo trial in surgery as patients usually know if they have or have not had an operation! However, in this study the patients who volunteered for the research were all given a general anaesthetic and all had surgical cuts in their knees. A third had joint lavage, a third had more sophisticated lavage in which they also had loose or torn cartilage removed by 'keyhole' surgical instruments inserted through the cuts and the last third were sewn up again without any treatment being done. Over two years of follow-up there was no difference in outcome – in fact the patients who had the 'dummy surgery' actually did fractionally better than the two treated groups. In the USA over 650,000 joint lavage operations are done annually, at a cost of over 1 billion dollars. For various reasons it is done proportionately less often in the UK but nonetheless it is difficult to escape the conclusion that joint lavage may be a useless treatment for OA.

STEROID INJECTIONS

Some trials have shown that injection of a steroid into the synovial fluid after removing the excess will dampen the inflammation (usually of the knee) and prolong the benefit. This probably works because steroids have powerful anti-inflammatory effects and once inside the knee joint they spread across and to some extent into the inflamed cartilage.

Even more care has to be taken to keep the procedure sterile when injecting steroid into a joint as steroid also dampens the body's immune response, so it is theoretically possible for infection to gain a firm hold in a steroid-treated joint. In practice this is a rare event. There is some worry that repeated steroid injections can speed up the wear process within a joint and so most doctors are cautious about repeating injections too often. There is no research information however on how many injections might be too much, or on what is the best spacing for repeat doses. (It is thought, however, that perhaps three such injections into any one joint in a year is unlikely to cause any damage.) The best judge is the individual person's response combined with common sense.

HYALURONIC ACID INJECTIONS

Hyaluronic acid has already been mentioned as a component of synovial fluid, and several trials have investigated the effectiveness of injecting it into the joint. Some results are favourable but others are less so and it is impossible to generalise. A proportion of people who have had hyaluronic acid injections get a temporary flare-up of their arthritis after the treatment. One can say that it is an option for people for whom surgery might be unsuitable or not desired, but with no guarantee of improvement.

Surgery

Undoubtedly the most dramatic development for joint arthritis in the past several decades has been the ability to replace all or part of the joint with an artificial component, or 'prosthesis'. It is now possible to replace shoulder, elbow, ankle and finger joints but the vast majority of joint replacements have been of the hip and the knee. The world's first joint replacements were conducted in the early 1960s by Sir John Charnley at Wrightington Hospital in Lancashire, following the development work on prototype artificial hips that he conducted in his garden shed.

Almost 80,000 major joint replacements are carried out annually in the UK and the demand for hip and knee replacement is estimated to increase by 40 per cent over the next 30 years due to the increase in numbers of elderly people in the population. Waiting lists for joint replacement in the NHS are lengthy and coping with this increase in need for surgery will be a major problem in the years ahead.

The decision on when it is appropriate to replace a joint with an artificial one is very much an individual one. The majority of people for whom joint replacement is done are those with severe pain and disability despite maximum medical treatment. The results of hip and knee replacement are excellent and most people get very good pain relief and improved mobility.

Artificial joints tend to work loose in time and so they have a limited lifespan before needing replacement. Artificial hips last 10–15 years or more; in fact 77 per cent of 'Charnley hips' are still functioning well 25 years later. Knee replacements are showing similar or better figures, with 90–95 per cent functioning at 10 years and over 90 per cent at 15 years. However, it can be difficult to replace an artificial joint and most surgeons therefore are reluctant to insert one in a young person unless it is absolutely necessary.

Complications of joint surgery are infrequent but some are potentially serious. One or two operations in every hundred are complicated by infection deep in the wound, which can require further surgery to put right. One operation in every 200 is associated with dislocation of the artificial joint, although this is rare for knee replacements and one in every 300 people will suffer a major clot in the veins (deep vein thrombosis or DVT) that dislodges and travels to the lung. Pulmonary embolism, as this is called, is a potentially fatal consequence of DVT but the risk of getting a DVT can be reduced by giving blood-thinning drugs around the time of the operation. Other risks are associated with a general anaesthetic for a major operation and because many people who have joint replacements are elderly these risks are higher than for operations more commonly done in younger people. About 1 per cent of people over 80 who have a joint replacement will suffer a heart attack or stroke related to the operation. Overall, one person in 200 dies following major joint replacement.

These figures may make joint replacement look more dangerous than it deserves. Much depends on the fitness of the person going for the surgery and careful assessment and preparation are now routine in UK orthopaedic centres. For many people with disabling arthritis a successful operation markedly improves their quality of life and makes the risks worth taking.

Key Points

- Osteoarthritis (OA) is a progressive disease of the cartilage of joints.
- OA is the commonest cause of joint pain in older people but it can also affect younger people, usually when there are other risk factors such as obesity or joint injury present.
- Treatments that significantly alter the rate at which OA develops are not yet available, so the treatment of OA aims to control pain and maintain or improve function in affected joints.
- Simple painkillers such as paracetamol or paracetamol/codeine combinations should be tried first.

- Non-steroidal anti-inflammatory drugs (NSAIDs) are also helpful and convenient painkillers in OA.
- Evidence for the effectiveness of 'cartilage protecting' drugs such as chondroitin and glucosamine is weak but they appear better than placebo and are generally safe.
- There is also some evidence in favour of several herbal remedies as painkillers in OA.
- Regular exercise helps to relieve pain and maintain function in OA.
- Physiotherapists can advise on the best types of exercise for an individual.
- Intervention treatments for OA range from the simple removal of excess synovial fluid, through injection of steroids or lubricating materials into the joint space to the replacement of severely arthritic joints.
- There is now doubt over the effectiveness of joint lavage – a commonly performed procedure on arthritic knees in particular.

Chapter 6

Non-steroidal Anti-inflammatory Drugs (NSAIDs)

Steroids and non-steroids

Inflammation is a general term in medicine that covers the body's response to injury, infection, auto-immune attack and many other situations. Steroids are hormones produced naturally by living beings and there are many of them, with different functions. Steroid drugs likewise come in different forms and with sometimes widely differing actions but in common medical usage the term steroid refers to a type of general purpose medicine that has powerful anti-inflammatory effects. Steroids are useful in literally hundreds of medical conditions including arthritis but they can be accompanied by many side effects, especially if they have to be used at a high dosage for a long time. These include salt retention, high blood pressure, weakening of the skin and bones, increased tendency to developing diabetes, stomach ulcers – and more.

The non-steroidal anti-inflammatory drugs attempt to obtain the desired effects of steroids, such as the anti-inflammatory property, but without all the side effects. To some extent they do achieve this. For example, they do not cause bone or skin weakening or increase the chance of getting diabetes. Unfortunately they can cause:

- bleeding from the digestive system (the commonest major side effect),
- raised blood pressure,
- allergic reactions and skin rashes,
- fluid retention.

Less common NSAID side effects include:

- **Asthma**: which can be triggered in people with an underlying tendency.
- **Kidney failure**: rarely this can occur and is usually reversible on stopping the drug. Kidney damage possibly occurs also to a small proportion of people who take NSAIDs at a high dose for years.

NSAID drugs have, over the years, come in for a lot of criticism, mainly because of their association with stomach ulcers and bleeding. It is worth emphasising though that they are effective analgesics and for many people with pain they are a lifeline. As we'll come to shortly, they can be used safely in a greater proportion of people by following some basic guidelines that rule out those at most risk of developing problems from the drugs.

Actions of NSAIDs

NSAIDs have three major actions:

1 REDUCTION OF INFLAMMATION
By this is meant the alleviation of local tissue changes that occur in a damaged or otherwise inflamed tissue, such as swelling and heat.

2 PAIN RELIEF

Mostly this is because they block the production by inflamed tissues of chemicals that cause pain.

3 LOWERING OF TEMPERATURE

NSAIDs seem to act on the 'thermostat' area within the brain to lower the temperature of the body in general when a fever is present. They do not lower a normal body temperature.

Over 50 NSAIDs have been discovered and more than 20 are available for prescription in the UK. Aspirin and paracetamol are technically NSAID drugs but are not officially classed within the group. Paracetamol has almost no anti-inflammatory properties in any case.

Ibuprofen is the benchmark NSAID against which others are usually measured and it is more fully described in appendix B. NSAIDs differ between each other in their tendency to cause side effects. There are probably also some relative differences in their effectiveness but there is little hard evidence for this in the medical literature. It is generally agreed that ibuprofen is the least likely to cause serious side effects on the digestive system but that it is a weaker anti-inflammatory than others. Medium risk NSAIDs are diclofenac, indometacin, ketoprofen, naproxen and piroxicam.

In practical terms all NSAIDs have the same possible side effects and the choice of which one to use is largely a process of trial and error. Every doctor tends to develop his or her own method of choosing these drugs for a patient and there is no best method. The most important issue about the use of NSAIDs is not which of them to use, but when to use them at all.

Minimising side effects from NSAIDs

Some people have a higher risk of developing side effects from NSAIDs and should either avoid the drugs or take extra steps to minimise the likelihood of problems occurring. Observing the following points will reduce the risks:

1 AVOID IN ULCER DISEASE OR 'INDIGESTION'

NSAIDs are not suitable for people with a history of stomach or duodenal ulcer. Certainly not if the ulcer is currently active and probably not if there is a history of a healed ulcer. People with a history of a bleeding ulcer are at particularly high risk of trouble from NSAIDs and should not use them, no matter how long ago they had the bleed. Indigestion should always be investigated if it lasts more than two or three weeks.

2 AVOID IN ELDERLY PEOPLE

People over 75 years are over five times more likely to develop a bleed from the digestive system due to a NSAID than someone under 65. A severe bleed can be life threatening at any age, but elderly people are again many times more likely to have a fatal bleed than a younger person. There are several reasons for this, including the fact that their bodies are less able to compensate for the blood loss, so they are more likely to suffer a severe drop in blood pressure, which in turn can more easily lead to a stroke or a heart attack for example.

3 CHOOSE THE SAFEST NSAID

Ibuprofen is the first choice as it has the least likelihood of causing bleeding. As for the other NSAIDs the evidence is less good that they are much safer, but diclofenac and naproxen are generally preferred. NSAID creams are effective in giving pain relief and, unlike the oral versions, they do not cause digestive upset.

4 USE AN ULCER-HEALING DRUG ALONG WITH THE NSAID

There is adequate evidence to show that a stomach-protecting drug called misoprostol, as well as an acid-reducing drug called omeprazole, are both effective at reducing the chance of ulcers arising from oral NSAID use. The results for omeprazole are superior. Using these drugs along with the NSAID reduces the chance of an ulcer arising, but does not remove it completely.

Other types of anti-ulcer drugs such as ranitidine and cimetidine do not protect against NSAID-induced ulcers in the doses normally used for healing ordinary ulcers but at double dosage they are protective.

There are some combination preparations available that combine misoprostol with either diclofenac or naproxen, but other than reducing the number of tablets needing to be swallowed they do not offer any extra advantages over separate medicines.

5 REMOVE *HELICOBACTER* INFECTION FROM THE STOMACH

Helicobacter pylori is the name of a bacterium that is very commonly found in the stomach lining of people with an ulcer of the stomach or duodenum (the outlet of the stomach). Eliminating *Helicobacter* with a short course of high-dose antibiotics and other drugs can dramatically improve the healing of such an ulcer, and prevent it coming back. There is some evidence to show that eliminating *Helicobacter* could be useful in reducing the chance of an NSAID-induced ulcer. There are several tests available to detect *Helicobacter*, the commonest and cheapest being a blood test to detect antibodies to the bug. If the blood test is positive then one assumes the person has been infected with *Helicobacter*, and gives the elimination treatment. Clearing *Helicobacter* from people taking NSAIDs is not done routinely and until more is known about its value it is probably best left as an option for a person at high risk of developing an ulcer but for whom NSAID treatment is effective and acceptable.

New NSAIDs

Prostaglandins, so called because they were first isolated from the prostate gland, are important hormone-like substances involved in a wide range of biological reactions in the body, including the process of inflammation. They are produced in many body tissues, including the lining of the digestive system, where they help protect the lining of the gut. (Misoprostol is in fact a synthetic prostaglandin, which accounts for its ulcer-healing property.) Prostaglandins are produced through the chemical actions of two enzymes called CoX-1 and CoX-2 and NSAIDs work because they switch off these CoX enzymes.

The CoX-2 enzyme produces prostaglandins involved most in the inflammatory process whereas the CoX-1 enzyme produces prostaglandins that protect the gut. In theory, therefore, it is only the CoX-2 enzyme that ought to be targeted. Older NSAIDs such as ibuprofen are, however, not selective, and switch off both CoX enzymes, which is why they reduce inflammation but also cause stomach ulcers.

Over the past few years several NSAIDs have been released which more selectively block the CoX-2 enzyme. They appear to be as effective as other NSAIDs in relieving the symptoms of arthritis and there is some evidence to suggest that they are less liable to cause bleeding from the gut.

There are five such NSAIDs currently available for arthritis: celecoxib, rofecoxib, meloxicam, etodolac and etoricoxib. GPs (in England and Wales officially but in fact throughout the UK) are expected to follow the guidance provided by the government's advisory body in prescribing matters, the National Institute for Clinical Excellence (NICE). NICE guidance states that it is not justified to transfer all prescriptions for NSAIDs to the CoX-2 types, mainly on cost grounds (an extra £45 million annually in the UK) and that instead the drugs should be used only in people at high risk of developing serious side effects such as bleeding. The high-risk groups examples are:

- people over 65 years,
- those also taking other medicines that can cause digestive upset,
- debilitated people,
- those taking maximum doses of NSAID drugs long term.

CoX-2 NSAIDs might reduce the chance of problems developing in someone with a past history of ulcers or bleeding from the gut but they are not free of risk. The use of any NSAID in such a person is therefore always a decision that needs to be made with care.

Taking aspirin, including low-dose aspirin as used by many people with heart disease for example, reduces or cancels the benefit of taking a CoX-2 NSAID, and there is not enough information yet available to say whether further gut protection can be had by adding a stomach-protecting drug to a CoX-2 NSAID.

Celecoxib currently has the most evidence in its favour as the NSAID least likely to cause stomach upset but CoX-2 NSAIDs are very much in the medical news at the time of writing (October 2002) and the debate is by no means over concerning their value.

Key Points

- NSAIDs are important and effective painkillers that can be used in OA as well as many other painful conditions.
- They can potentially cause significant side effects such as ulcers or bleeding from the digestive system.
- The risks of complications arising from NSAIDs can be minimised by avoiding their use in high-risk patients and by using strategies to protect the stomach.
- There is little or no difference in the effectiveness of the commonly used NSAIDs but small differences in their side effects can make it worth trying an alternative if the first choice causes unwanted symptoms.
- CoX-2 NSAIDs are a newer group that are less likely to cause digestive upset. They are recommended for use only in people with higher risk of developing such side effects.
- Aspirin reduces or cancels any protective effect from a CoX-2 NSAID.

Chapter 7

Rheumatoid Arthritis

The classification of arthritis into types that are either 'inflammatory' or 'degenerative' is based on whether the immune system (i.e. the process of inflammation) is thought to play a part in causing the condition. Although this is a useful and still commonly used way of grouping the many different forms of arthritis it is not strictly accurate. Osteoarthritis, for example, is the commonest degenerative form, but it is now understood to be more complex than just 'wear and tear' of the joints and almost certainly involves the immune system in some ways too.

'Inflammatory arthritis' is an umbrella term for dozens of distinct joint diseases but some of these are quite rare. Rheumatoid arthritis is by far the commonest inflammatory type and is the main one discussed in this book. Information on some others is presented in the following chapters.

What is rheumatoid arthritis?

Rheumatoid arthritis (RA) is a disease primarily of the synovial lining (synovium) of joints (chapter 1). Initially the synovium seems to be stimulated to overgrow. It thickens, sometimes quite markedly, so that extra folds of synovium build up within the joint space and strands of extra tissue float in the synovial fluid like seaweed. Numerous cells that are members of the body's immune system build up within the abnormal synovium. At the edges of the synovium the synovial cells migrate in towards the joint cartilage, slowly eroding and destroying it in the process. This is helped by the release of enzymes from the inflammatory cells that by now are in high numbers throughout the synovium and which break down the cartilage. Where muscles are attached to bones by tendons there is also synovial tissue, which can also be affected in RA. Thus RA typically affects many of the tissues surrounding joints, and not just the lining cartilage. In fact RA is associated with many complications of tissues other than the joints, hence rheumatologists usually refer to it more generally as 'rheumatoid disease' rather than rheumatoid arthritis alone.

Such non-joint problems include small lumps under the skin, called rheumatoid nodules, that are commonest at pressure points such as the elbows, forearms, wrists and feet. Others are inflammation of the tissues that cover the lungs and heart, abnormalities within lung tissue, dryness of the eyes and anaemia to name a few. Why these extra problems arise in RA is unknown, as there is no synovial tissue in the affected places. As with OA, much remains to be understood in RA.

Features of rheumatoid arthritis

Of more practical importance is what effects all these underlying changes have on someone with the condition.

JOINTS

RA is a disease in which many joints become affected at the same time. In the early stages this might be some of the small joints of the hands and feet but larger weight-bearing joints such as the knee and hip can also be involved. The knuckle joints of the hands (MCP joints) or the next joint out in the fingers (PIP joints) are the most typical to be inflamed and swollen and often the wrists are sore. In the feet the commonest affected joints are those at the bases of the toes – those you stand on when you take the weight off your heels (MTP joints).

Someone with RA will notice that in the morning the affected joints are a bit stiff and they take a while to ease off. This is due to synovial fluid having built up in the inflamed joints overnight but which clears a bit during the day. In the early stages of RA these might be all the symptoms that are present. With the improvements in treatment for RA that now exist many more people have worsening of their arthritis prevented over the ensuing years. However RA cannot yet be cured, and many people do eventually suffer more advanced forms of the condition.

These result from the progressive attack on the joints of the inflamed synovial tissues and the additional effects on the muscles and tendons surrounding the joints. The tendons that move across the surfaces of the fingers slip off to the side, pulling the fingers into a curled position and also swinging them at the MCP joints in the direction of the little finger. Quite often the tendons slip off completely at some of the small finger joints and give rise to characteristic angular deformities of the fingers. Naturally this compromises grip strength and dexterity. Inflammation of the tendons gives rise to pain in the hands and wrists. RA in the toes makes them curl and puts pressure on the MTP joints on walking. This can be very uncomfortable but can be helped a lot by specially fitted shoes.

SPINE

Although RA affects mostly the joints of the limbs it does also affect the spine in a number of recognised patterns. Each of the main joints between the vertebrae and the spongy shock-absorbing 'discs' is of a different type to the synovial joints but throughout the spine there are extensive attachments of muscles and tendons, all of which are vulnerable to the process of RA. Slippage can occur in the alignment of the vertebrae and this can put pressure on the spinal cord. Spinal cord pressure gives rise to problems with the function of the nerves connected to the spinal cord at that level and, if severe, to the rest of the spinal cord below the level of compression. This causes weakness of the muscles to which the nerves are connected as well as pain or altered sensation. A complication that is fortunately rare but is characteristic for RA is slippage between the top vertebra in the neck (called the atlas) and the one below it (the axis). This can put potentially dangerous pressure on the spinal cord as the atlas slips forward on top of the axis on bending the neck forward. Surgery is required to stabilise the neck in this condition and may be required to relieve nerve pressure in less dangerous but nonetheless troublesome examples of cord or nerve pressure elsewhere along the spine.

NERVE TRAPPING

Less serious and commoner problems can arise when nerves are trapped in regions away from the spinal cord itself. There are three common points for this to occur – at the wrist, elbow and ankle.

1 **Wrist**: within the wrist, in a space called the carpal tunnel that is just a few square centimetres in cross section, are packed the small bones of the wrist and the ends of the two main forearm bones, the multiple tendons and muscles to control the fingers, arteries taking blood to the hand and veins taking blood away, three main nerves to control the muscles within the hand and carry the signals of sensation plus various support and strengthening tissues, fat and skin. In short, there is no spare room! Swelling of the synovial tendon coverings here therefore compresses the structures and one nerve in particular, called the median nerve, which runs through the middle of the wrist. This causes pain, tingling and numbness in the

area that the median nerve goes to. This generally is to the palm side of the thumb plus the index and long fingers and the adjacent part of the ring finger, but there is some variation in this pattern between different people. Typically the symptoms waken the person from sleep, and they get relief by shaking their hand about. This condition, called carpal tunnel syndrome, can also be caused by several conditions other than RA.

2 **Elbow**: two major nerves that curve round the elbow joint can be trapped in their course here. The ulnar nerve fits in to a groove on the inside of the elbow (the 'funny bone') and if compressed causes elbow pain and numbness down the inside of the forearm (in medicine the convention is to refer to the position of the arm when it is held by the side with the palm facing forward). The radial nerve runs through the front of the elbow and if it is compressed here there will be pain in the forearm on cocking back the wrist or the fingers, as this stretches the nerve. If uncorrected it can cause the wrist to droop due to muscle weakness.

3 **Ankle**: a problem similar to ulnar nerve trapping can occur on the inside of the ankle and cause pain and numbness on the inside of the foot.

As with spinal compression, surgery can be required for any of these trapped nerve syndromes if they are severe enough. In carpal tunnel syndrome a less invasive remedy that can work is to inject a steroid into the wrist at the carpal tunnel, which has the effect of reducing inflammation and swelling. The improvement, if any, may however be only temporary.

OTHER PROBLEMS

People with active RA often feel generally tired. This can be just a general sign of activity of the immune system – for example when fighting off a dose of the 'flu' it's common to feel quite fatigued. In RA, however, there can also be a degree of anaemia (blood lack) caused either by the arthritis or as a side effect of some of the medicines used to treat it. If pain from inflamed joints is not adequately controlled then sleep may be poor, which leads to daytime fatigue.

Dry eyes are quite commonly seen alongside RA, due to deficient tear production. There are numerous other recognised features of RA that tend to be seen only in more severe or longstanding disease. One such is the inflammation of very small arteries in the fingers and toes that can reduce the blood flow through them. This can cause ulcers in the skin. Weakness of the bones due to osteoporosis (chapter 11) can occur in RA both as a direct result of the condition and because steroid drugs, often used to treat RA, themselves cause bone thinning as a side effect. One of the many reasons that it is essential for anyone with RA to see a rheumatology specialist regularly is to ensure that these various aspects of the condition are looked for and monitored and that corrective action is taken whenever possible.

Some of the other findings such as laboratory test results and X-rays are covered later in this chapter, along with more detail on how a doctor makes the diagnosis of RA.

How common is rheumatoid arthritis?

Rheumatoid arthritis affects about 1 per cent of the adult population, so it is about twenty times less common than OA. About 12,000 people are newly diagnosed with RA each year in the UK.

Slightly more women than men get RA and there is a trend downwards over the past 40 to 50 years in the numbers of people affected. The reasons for the fall are unknown. One theory is that the oral contraceptive pill has a protective effect against the development of RA in women but this is uncertain.

RA is commoner in older people but can appear at any age. For every one person between 16 and 44 affected there are nine in the age range 45–64 and 12 aged 65 or over. Children under 16 can get it too, when it is called 'juvenile idiopathic' or 'juvenile rheumatoid' arthritis. Currently this affects about 12,000 children in the UK.

There is no evidence that RA differs in frequency across the regions of the UK but there is some evidence to say that people with RA who are from socially deprived areas have a poorer outcome. RA is less common in people of Pakistani or Afro-Caribbean origin than Caucasians.

Causes of rheumatoid arthritis

The general factors that are known to be important in causing arthritis were covered in chapter 2. A great deal of information is now known about RA but a single factor that triggers it has not been found. It seems more likely that RA is a destination that can be reached by different roads and that there are individual factors that determine its cause in any one person.

GENES
RA tends to be commoner among family members, which indicates that there is some genetic factor in its cause. Genes are the units of information that are stored in their thousands on the chromosomes within our cells, and are themselves comprised of collections of DNA. Each gene contains the necessary information for the manufacture and control of a protein molecule that may in turn take part in any one or more of the huge numbers of chemical and biological actions that occur continuously in the body. Some medical conditions are due to single 'faults' in an individual gene, but this is not so in RA. There appear to be many different combinations of gene types that can influence an individual's likelihood of developing RA. The potential combinations are so complex and numerous that very few patterns have been found that reliably predict whether someone will get RA. Some of the genetic 'markers' are, however, known to indicate the severity of the RA rather than the cause.

ENVIRONMENT
A person's genetic make-up is like an outline sketch on top of which life events paint the colours. Increasingly it is observed that it is the

combination of environment and susceptibility that determines whether someone gets a particular disease. This is equally seen in diabetes, asthma, high blood pressure, various forms of cancer – in fact perhaps all illnesses are thus determined. The environmental trigger can take any number of forms such as diet, exposure to chemicals or irritants, infection, psychological stress, and so on.

Infection is a good candidate as the trigger factor for RA, but again we don't have a single candidate to blame. Probably many virus or bacterial infections are potentially able to start off the process that ultimately leads to RA. Diet information is inconsistent as far as cause is concerned but fish oils might have a *protective* role against RA. Smoking might increase someone's chance of getting RA and/or increase the chance of more active disease.

Diagnosing rheumatoid arthritis

The appearance of the joints in someone who has had active RA for a long time is quite easy to recognise but what one wants to do is to recognise the disease at an early stage, so that active treatment can be established before too much joint damage has occurred. Unlike osteo-arthritis, in which very little can be done to halt its progress, rheumatoid arthritis can be slowed down considerably. This has led to the modern approach to RA treatment, which involves the introduction of 'disease modifying anti-rheumatic drugs' ('DMARDs' for short) at an early stage.

Making an early diagnosis is, however, more difficult because the available information is less definite – a bit like putting together a jigsaw puzzle with lots of missing pieces and only a part of the picture on the box to guide you.

A checklist widely used by specialists is the American College of Rheumatology diagnostic criteria which lists seven points, four of which need to be present for at least six weeks for rheumatoid arthritis to be diagnosed:

1 Morning stiffness of joints lasting at least an hour.
2 At least three joints affected.

3 Arthritis of hand joints (wrist, MCP or PIP).
4 Symmetrical arthritis, i.e. the equivalent joint in each limb.
5 Skin nodules.
6 Positive blood test for 'rheumatoid factor' (see below).
7 Recognised X-ray changes of RA seen in the bones of the hands or wrists.

In real life the diagnosis is, of course, harder than ticking items on a check sheet and it can be difficult for any doctor to be sure. Most GPs will defer the diagnosis to a rheumatologist but they can arrange for some common tests prior to the referral that are useful in screening for RA, and the specialist will probably use several more to diagnose the arthritis precisely and help guide treatment. Although much of this information is very detailed and best left to the specialist to interpret, some of the main points are worth knowing if you have RA – or indeed any type of arthritis. Some of the other relevant information on making a diagnosis of arthritis is in chapter 4.

Tests for rheumatoid arthritis

BLOOD TESTS
Rheumatoid factor is an antibody present in the blood of 75 per cent or more of people with RA and can be present years before someone develops any of the symptoms or signs of the condition. Unfortunately it is also commonly found in other auto-immune diseases and even in many people who remain completely healthy throughout their lives. 20–25 per cent of people with definite RA are negative for rheumatoid factor, so its limitations are obvious. High amounts of rheumatoid factor do, however, tend to be associated with very active RA.

X-RAYS
In chapter 4 we mentioned that X-rays were rarely of much use in diagnosing arthritis. In osteoarthritis, for example, they generally tell a doctor what he or she already knows simply by examining the patient.

In RA, however, they can be of more value because some of the features that are detectable by X-ray are not visible to the naked eye on examining the joint. One of the most important features of this type is what looks like a small hole in the bone next to an affected joint. The jargon term for this is an 'erosion' and they are seen earliest in the hands or feet.

OTHER TESTS

Modern technology has produced several other types of machine capable of producing images of joints. High frequency sound waves called ultrasound have been with us now for decades and are familiar to most mothers who have had a baby in recent years. Ultrasound works a bit like radar by bouncing the sound off the structures underneath the skin and analysing the reflections that come back and it is particularly good at detecting different densities of fluid. High resolution ultrasound (HRUS) is capable of very detailed pictures of joints and can pick up small effusions (collections of excess synovial fluid within joints) and swelling of synovial tissue. Presently the use of HRUS in the UK is severely limited by NHS funding restrictions but it is proving to be a useful tool for rheumatology specialists in the better funded health care systems of most of the rest of Europe.

MRI (magnetic resonance imaging) is a technique based on the fact that human beings are mostly made of water (admittedly this is a simplification!). In an MRI scan the patient lies within a magnetic field and then radio pulses are rapidly switched on and off. This causes the water molecules of the body to 'resonate' and in doing so emit their own radio signal, which the machine detects and translates into an image. MRI is particularly good at giving detailed images of the fine structure within joints and within the spinal canal if spinal cord compression is suspected.

Technology, it has to be said, cannot alone diagnose RA or any other type of arthritis. It provides useful extra information but most of the time it is the skill of the physician in clarifying the pattern of the arthritis combined with the findings on simple examination and easily available tests that are the important elements of making an accurate diagnosis.

Assessment of function

Giving a disease a name is only part of the purpose of making a diagnosis. Particularly important in joint disease is the effect it has upon a person's ability to carry out the daily tasks of life, so an assessment of someone's abilities should be part of routine care. There are many different ways to do this, from observing someone going about their house to asking them to complete standardised questionnaires on the difficulties they are having, if any. The method used is less important than the fact that it is done at all. In the UK occupational therapists are the professional group most involved in this aspect of care and they are likely to have been involved with most or all people with severe arthritis or who have been seen by a specialist in rheumatology. It is worth bearing in mind that many other people with perhaps less severe arthritis could benefit from their advice.

Aims of treatment

Put simply, treating RA ought to make someone feel better, but there are more organised criteria than this. Along the same lines as the diagnostic checklist the American College of Rheumatology lists six points, the presence of five of which for two months or more will count as a remission of the disease. Remission implies that the arthritis is dormant rather than completely cured – as yet we have no treatment that can achieve the latter goal.

The list is:

1 Morning stiffness present for a maximum of 15 minutes.
2 No fatigue.
3 No joint pain.
4 No joint tenderness or pain on moving joints.

5 No swelling of joints or around them.

6 ESR reading (chapter 4) below 30 for women and 20 for men.

Remission in these terms will of, course, automatically mean that the person will feel better, but it is recognised that the list is difficult to achieve. Technology might also help to determine when treatment is working and when it is not – MRI or HRUS might prove useful here but this is an area of research study and not yet established within RA treatment in general.

The importance of this is not just academic. First, we know that RA can be active in joints that otherwise do not appear inflamed, so a person's symptoms cannot be used as the sole guide to whether treatment is effective. Somewhere down the line an inflamed joint will give trouble again, even if it is presently not doing so. Second, several of the drugs used in RA treatment are potentially capable of causing significant side effects, so we need to be able to monitor the progress of RA in detail if we are to make worthwhile judgements on whether the risks of treatment are worthwhile. Ideally a system of repeated functional assessment combined with the results of specialist examination and laboratory tests should be routine for all patients receiving the best care for their RA. This is particularly relevant when it comes to the proper use of the most recent drugs developed for use in RA, which act directly on the immune system. More details of these are at the end of this chapter.

Non-drug treatment

The broadest classification of the treatment of RA is into non-drug and drug-based therapies. As with life in general, it is the simple things that can matter the most. If someone with bad arthritis of the weight-bearing joints is too heavy then they will benefit from weight loss. If a wrist is particularly inflamed and sore then a strap-on wrist support will help. If someone has active arthritis of the feet with clawing of the toes then custom-fitted shoes will be more comfortable than standard mass-produced ones. If a person is going through a period when their arthritis is particularly active then they will benefit from rest, which might require a spell off work. Tight taps can be operated more easily with lever extensions and weakened muscles can be built up with exercise programmes.

This is all common sense and it is to be hoped that all people with RA are already advised well along these lines. Those who feel they are not should discuss the matter with their GP or specialist.

SURGERY

Surgery for RA is a particularly specialised field and orthopaedic surgeons who have an interest in this work co-operate closely with rheumatology specialist physicians, occupational therapists, physiotherapists and foot specialists (podiatrists) to achieve the best results. Technically it is feasible to replace almost any synovial joint and some of the most dramatic improvements in function can be obtained by replacing diseased finger joints for example.

Joint replacement is, however, not the only operative choice for someone with RA. Sometimes the surgeon will need only to do a smaller operation, such as the movement of a tendon, to make a big difference to someone's ability to use their hand. Removal of excess synovial tissues from inflamed tendon sheaths at the wrist can prevent the underlying tendons from rupturing – a known complication of RA. These sorts of operation are therefore done in advance of further problems arising. Successful joint surgery requires good teamwork between the professionals involved, good communication with the patient and a clear understanding in advance of what will be achieved by it. Fortunately, in the NHS the level of specialist advice and skill is very high.

Drug treatment

Doctors have largely regarded RA as a condition that one treats with drugs, and for good reasons. Some medications undoubtedly slow the progress or limit the activity of RA, in contrast to the situation with OA which largely takes its own course, with a few exceptions (chapter 5).

Many of the details of the drug treatment of RA are highly technical and somewhat bewildering to the non-specialist doctor, let alone an interested member of the general public, but the broad principles can be summarised.

Historically, the medical approach has been to use ordinary painkillers and NSAIDs for early RA, in the same way as with osteoarthritis and then move on to the more 'powerful' drugs (DMARDs) as the disease progressed or for those people whose symptoms were hard to control with simple measures. The modern approach is to use DMARDs early in the hope that this will brake the progress of RA.

NSAIDS

NSAID use is covered in chapter 6 and there are no particular aspects of it in RA that are any different. NSAIDs have no effect upon the progress of RA.

STEROID DRUGS

Sometimes the injection of a special steroid solution into a joint affected by osteoarthritis will give temporary relief of symptoms but otherwise steroids do not help OA. In rheumatoid arthritis however not only are such joint injections useful but oral steroid has been and remains one of the most important main treatments.

'Steroid' is in fact a general term for a host of different proteins produced within the body and many more artificial ones invented by drug companies that have a wide range of different effects. The types of steroid used in treating RA, and in other medical applications, are called corticosteroids and they have the ability to dampen down the action of the immune system. Natural corticosteroids are produced by the adrenal glands, which are two walnut-sized pieces of specialised tissue that sit on top of each kidney.

Steroids are usually used in tablet form, but there are several different preparations available, including long-lasting injections. They all have the same pattern of benefits and side effects, which are increased in proportion to the dosage.

Steroids usually work very quickly and can calm down active arthritis within just a few days. Having achieved this effect the aim is then to reduce the dose as much and as rapidly as possible to avoid the side effects – which are many. Steroids thin the skin (causing easy bruising) and weaken the bone structure (causing osteoporosis). They increase body weight and cause fluid retention, raise the blood pressure and the likelihood of developing diabetes, predispose to developing cataracts in the lenses of the eyes and can cause ulcers and bleeding from the stomach and digestive system – and this is not a complete list. With such a fearful stack of potential problems one might wonder why they ever get used but the positive side is that they can work wonders in a short time in someone crippled by very active inflammatory arthritis. That also means that they can be hard to stop unless the arthritis is dampened by other treatment capable of doing so but which is not steroid based.

The commonest prescribed oral steroid in the UK is prednisolone. As a rough guide a daily dose of prednisolone below 10 milligrams (mg) is considered a low dose and will cause relatively few side effects. 50 mg daily or even more might be required to control a very active arthritis but would cause many of the listed side effects within just a few weeks. It is common to have to make a compromise with steroid treatment between effectively dampening the arthritis and avoiding too many side effects of treatment.

Additional measures other than dose reduction that can be taken to minimise the problems of steroid therapy include:

Bone protection
Drugs to stimulate bone growth are used to treat osteoporosis (chapter 11) and are now standard (or should be) in anyone taking long-term steroid treatment. Bone loss from steroids occurs particularly in the first few months, so protection should be considered right away in anyone needing steroid treatment that is likely to last for this length of time. The effects on bone strength can be measured periodically by

bone scans but provision of the necessary equipment in the UK is currently inadequate to do this for everyone who needs it.

Gut protection

Anti-ulcer drugs were mentioned in chapter 6 as being helpful in reducing the likelihood of developing ulcers or gut bleeding from NSAIDs. Whether they do the same for steroid therapy is less certain, but some experts recommend them. As many or most people taking steroids will also be taking an NSAID then the case for using stomach-protecting drugs alongside is stronger. Elimination of *Helicobacter* infection is also recommended for the same reasons as previously covered.

An important aspect of long-term steroid treatment is that it must not be stopped suddenly. Doing so not only allows the underlying condition for which it is being used to flare up right away, but can expose the person to a potentially dangerous drop in the general steroid levels in the body. This is because the adrenal glands effectively shut down their own steroid production when artificial steroids are being taken. Although adrenal gland activity recovers when external steroids are withdrawn they do so slowly, and for a while the amount of steroid in the body drops too low for the many biological processes in which they are used. In the most severe cases this can cause collapse. By withdrawing steroids slowly, usually over some weeks, the adrenal glands have time to become fully functional again

Disease-modifying anti-rheumatic drugs (DMARDs)

This is where RA treatment gets particularly complex. Not only are there several groups of DMARDs, but it is possible to combine them and it requires considerable expertise to judge the best treatment for an individual person. They also have a wide range of possible side effects, many of them potentially quite serious although this should not prevent their use – they can be used safely under proper guidance. In this book only a general guide can be given. Some of the main side effects of each group of drugs are listed here and more are in appendix B but it has to be emphasised that these lists are incomplete and they should not be relied on when making any decision on a choice or change of treatment.

DMARDs do not act as painkillers but they dampen the inflammation of RA and thereby reduce the symptoms gradually. It is usual for them to take many weeks to begin to work, which is important to bear in mind when starting treatment. Not much is really understood about how any of the DMARDs actually work. Most were discovered by good fortune and careful observation of people with RA who were given the drugs for completely different reasons and coincidentally were noted to have improvement in their arthritis.

METHOTREXATE

Methotrexate blocks the duplication of cells and so is a widely used anti-cancer drug. How it works in RA is not understood, but it has a powerful dampening effect on RA and is now commonly used as the first choice DMARD. Methotrexate must be given only once per week to avoid adverse effects upon the bone marrow, which is the site of production of the various cells that are present in blood. It can also cause liver inflammation and kidney damage. Regular checks on the blood are therefore necessary. Before starting methotrexate most rheumatologists arrange for the patient to have a chest X-ray and lung check, as the drug can, rarely, cause inflammation and scarring of the lungs (this would show as a cough and breathlessness). More common are small sores of the mouth. Despite these potential problems most people tolerate methotrexate quite well.

SULFASALAZINE

Sulfasalazine is a combination of salicylate (the active ingredient in aspirin) with another compound that is split off by the action of bacteria in the gut. The salicylate is then absorbed and exerts its anti-inflammatory effects on the arthritis. The main side effects of sulfasalazine are digestive upset and headache but adverse effects on the red and white cells of the blood can occur. Regular blood checks are therefore necessary.

ANTI-MALARIAL DRUGS

Chloroquine and its related compound hydroxychloroquine have been around for decades as treatments for malaria. They can take three or four months to show a response in RA. Both drugs can cause damage to the light-sensitive part of the eye (the retina) but hydroxychloroquine is much less likely to do so than chloroquine. As there is no difference in the results of treatment between the two drugs, chloroquine is probably best abandoned. Periodic eye checks are still recommended when using hydroxychloroquine.

IMMUNE SYSTEM SUPPRESSING DRUGS

There are several drugs in this group, methotrexate being one too, but these others are used less often. Examples are:

- Leflunomide
- Ciclosporin
- Cyclophosphamide

GOLD COMPOUNDS

Twenty to 30 years ago gold compounds were the main DMARDs in use but they are now less popular. They take several months to begin working and are associated with skin rashes, mouth ulcers, blood disturbance and kidney damage, which shows first as the appearance of protein in the urine. Blood and urine checks are therefore required regularly.

D-PENICILLAMINE

Like gold salts, penicillamine is now outmoded, although not yet obsolete. It has similar effects and side effects to gold and also requires careful monitoring. Penicillamine can be made by chemically splitting penicillin, the antibiotic, hence the similar name.

BIOLOGICAL AGENTS

Research into the causes of rheumatoid arthritis combined with the rapid expansion of knowledge and techniques available in bio-technology has led to a number of new types of treatment. These are all proteins that act in some way or other upon the cells or processes that take part in inflammation. Tumour necrosis factor (TNF), for example, is a substance produced naturally by the 'clearing-up' cells of the immune system but is produced in excess in RA. TNF activates the inflammatory process, so blocking its effect reduces the amount of inflammation. Two drugs are available which can block TNF:

1 Etanercept
2 Infliximab

Both of these drugs are expensive and their accepted use within the NHS is subject to the guidance of NICE (National Institute for Clinical Excellence). They should be used only after failure of treatment with at least two other DMARDs, including methotrexate. Serious reactions that can occur with these drugs include nervous system damage, blood disturbance and infections such as tuberculosis. Infliximab has to be strictly avoided in pregnancy and has to be given with methotrexate. Despite such potential problems these drugs are important advances in the range of treatment available for RA. They effectively dampen active disease in the majority of people to whom they are given and reduce the general feelings of ill health and fatigue that can accompany it. We do not yet have long-term studies to indicate how they will behave over the course of many years. Anakinra is another biological agent now available for use in RA and many other such compounds are being studied.

Use of DMARDs

Clearly the use of DMARDs is complicated, and not without potential hazard. They are always used under specialist supervision, but for someone with active RA they can make the disease very much more tolerable. In practice, problems occur less frequently than it may appear from reading the rather daunting lists of possible side effects. One of the many skills needed by the specialist in rheumatology is to match the strength of treatment to the activity of the individual's arthritis, and to minimise the ill effects of treatment by careful dosage, combining DMARDs where required. Unlike some other clinical problems, such as high blood pressure, there are no definite guidelines on how best to treat rheumatoid arthritis. Each person requires skilled individual assessment and long-term care and should feel an equal partner in treatment decisions. Clear explanations of the risks and benefits of any treatment are essential and the best results are always obtained where there has been good co-operation between all parties.

Key Points

- Rheumatoid arthritis is the commonest inflammatory arthritis, affecting about 1 per cent of the population.
- The inflamed synovial tissues in RA progressively attack and destroy the cartilage within affected joints.
- RA is probably caused by environmental triggers in individuals who have a genetic tendency to develop the condition, but this area of knowledge is very incomplete.
- Diagnosis rests on a combination of clinical features and laboratory tests. High amounts of rheumatoid factor in the blood are associated with more active arthritis.

- Non-drug treatments include rest and splinting of inflamed joints, adequate pain relief, physiotherapy and exercise, customised footwear and other appliances as required.
- Surgery in RA includes joint replacement when necessary but also smaller interventions that preserve or improve function.
- Non-steroidal anti-inflammatory drugs and other painkillers are as useful in RA as in any other type of arthritis.
- Steroids, by mouth or injected into joints, can be used to quickly dampen active arthritis but higher doses are accompanied by significant side effects in the long term.
- The progress of RA can be slowed by disease-modifying anti-rheumatic drugs (DMARDs) and modern treatment uses DMARDs early to prevent joint damage.
- Powerful new treatments for RA have been developed and more are in the pipeline for the future.

Chapter 8

Other Inflammatory Joint Conditions

There are dozens of other types of arthritis and space is too limited to cover them. For most, the general principles of treatment that have been outlined for OA and RA also apply. Non-steroidal drugs generally work just as well in all forms of arthritis at relieving pain and stiffness and DMARDs may also be used in treating some, although not always with the same results seen in RA.

Three main examples are covered here:

1 Ankylosing spondylitis (the main condition in the group, exact cause unknown).
2 Reiter's syndrome (arthritis triggered by preceding gut or genital infection).
3 Psoriatic arthritis (associated with the skin condition called psoriasis).

A technical term often used to cover these is 'spondyloarthropathies'.

The prefix 'spondylo' means 'to do with the spine', which is the characteristic site at which these types of arthritis are active. However, the spondyloarthropathies also have some other features in common:

- They involve the joints at either side of the base of the spine, where the spine joins the wing-shaped pelvic bones (these are the sacro-iliac joints).
- Other small joints are also involved as well as those where the tendons of muscles are attached to the bones (for example Achilles tendonitis, which is a painful swelling at the back of the heel where the Achilles tendon joins the heel bone to the calf muscle above).
- Other tissues can be involved, such as the eye (iritis), lungs and heart.
- Rheumatoid factor is absent in these types of arthritis, which gives rise to another medical jargon term used to describe them as 'seronegative'.
- The HLA type B27 is present to a variable degree among them, the highest being in whites affected by ankylosing spondylitis, in whom over 95 per cent are B27 positive.

Ankylosing spondylitis

The word 'ankylosis' is the medical term for 'fusion', and in advanced ankylosing spondylitis (AS) the main finding is that the adjacent vertebrae of the spine become stiffly linked together. This reduces the flexibility of the spine considerably and can cause a bowing forward of the spine so that the affected person stoops markedly. Many people with AS do not however develop such severe changes and modern treatment minimises the chance of developing spinal deformity.

AS is nearly three times more common in men and in certain ethnic groups such as some Inuit and North American Indian tribes. It occurs in about 0.2–1 per cent of the white population in the UK.

FEATURES OF ANKYLOSING SPONDYLITIS

The symptoms that should suggest AS include:

- ache in the buttocks or base of the spine that is worse after inactivity and gets better after exercise,
- fatigue,
- persistence of these symptoms for more than three months.

Other pointers that make AS the likely diagnosis would be:

- family history of AS,
- age below 40 years,
- Achilles tendonitis or other conditions in which ligaments or tendons are inflamed, such as rib discomfort on breathing (costochondritis) or pains in the sole of the foot (plantar fasciitis),
- inflammation of the front of the eye (iritis). This shows as sudden pain and redness of the eyes and blurring of vision. Eye symptoms should always be assessed urgently by a doctor.

There are many other possible features of AS, including weight loss, poor appetite, arthritis of the limb joints (which tends to be seen more often in women), angina and breathlessness from inflammation of the heart arteries among others but these would be more likely to be present in the later stages of the condition.

DIAGNOSING ANKYLOSING SPONDYLITIS

On clinical examination several points might be observed by the doctor, the most useful being limited movement of the spine. This can be seen, for example, by observing someone's lower spine from behind and then getting them to bend forward. On careful observation one can see that the distance between the bony points that mark each of the vertebrae gets slightly greater on bending as the normally flexible spine bends. However, this does not happen if the spine is stiff, and the person instead bends from the hip with the spine staying straight.

X-ray of the spine is the most important test as this will show characteristic changes in the sacro-iliac joints and possibly also in the vertebrae. In someone with very early AS the spine X-rays might be normal, in which case the diagnosis could only be provisional. Repeating the X-rays some weeks or months later would then show the changes to confirm the diagnosis.

MRI scanning of the sacro-iliac joints can be very useful in early or mild AS as it can show up changes not seen on ordinary X-rays. Additionally MRI scanning uses very little radiation, which is an important consideration especially in younger or female patients.

Blood tests are of little value. Although the HLA-B27 test is likely to be positive one would not make a diagnosis of AS on this test alone. HLA-B27 is present in about 10 per cent of the general UK population so there is a fair chance that it would be positive in someone who does not have AS. By definition, rheumatoid factor is absent from the blood of someone with AS.

TREATMENT

The early symptoms of morning stiffness and pain respond well to ordinary painkillers or NSAIDs. Exercise is very important to maintain flexibility and itself relieves the symptoms, so good advice from a physiotherapist is invaluable as well as motivation on the part of the patient to keep themselves active on a regular basis. Swimming is an excellent form of exercise that maintains mobility in all of the joints.

Methotrexate and sulfasalazine are the two most common DMARDs in use for AS but the spinal arthritis responds less well to drug treatment than inflammation of the limb joints. Steroids in high dose can help sudden flare-ups of AS but they are of no value in longer-term use. The new 'biological agents' are currently being researched in AS and there is initial evidence to suggest that they are beneficial.

Weakening of the bones (osteoporosis) is more commonly seen in AS than in the average population, so medicines to protect against it are often also prescribed. Associated problems such as iritis usually occur independently of how active the arthritis is, and require treatment by an eye specialist. Steroid eye drops are usually used to dampen episodes of iritis and they work well.

Like RA, ankylosing spondylitis is not a curable condition but it can be well controlled. The general outlook for someone with the condition is excellent and there are good prospects for better treatment in the near future.

Reiter's syndrome

It has long been noticed that inflammatory arthritis can follow a number of different types of infection. Usually these are either gut infections (gastroenteritis) or infections of the genital system. It seems that some types of organism can trigger a reaction in the immune system of susceptible people, which then results in arthritis, although the organisms themselves are not present in the inflamed joint. There are quite a few terms and definitions used to describe different sub-types within this group (such as 'reactive arthritis') but the main condition is Reiter's syndrome.

Reiter's syndrome occurs in both sexes but is more common in men. Several of the bacteria well known to cause food poisoning, such as *Salmonella* and *Campylobacter*, are the likeliest to cause the gut type and *Chlamydia trachomatis* is the organism most likely to cause the sexually transmitted form. Interestingly some protein components of the *Chlamydia* organism have been detected within the affected joints of people with Reiter's syndrome even though the bug cannot be grown from samples taken from the joint.

The typical features of Reiter's syndrome are of inflammation of one or two joints in the lower limbs (knee, ankle or MTP joints) plus a history of gut or genital infection in the preceding six weeks or so. Occasionally the initial infection causes little or no symptoms, and the fact that it has happened is revealed only after laboratory tests have been done. Inflammation of the urethra (urine channel) can occur in either sex and gives rise to discomfort passing urine. In women inflammation of the cervix can cause discomfort or discharge from the vagina. (Note: these genital problems can occur from Reiter's syndrome that has been triggered by *either* a gut or a genital infection.)

The additional features, not all of which might be present, reflect the overlap between this and ankylosing spondylitis:

- fever,
- fatigue,
- sacro-iliac pain,
- skin rash,
- eye inflammation.

Treatment of Reiter's syndrome is along the same lines as for AS although steroid treatment, both as oral therapy and/or as injections into inflamed joints, is more useful than in AS. About half of people with Reiter's syndrome develop repeated attacks.

Safe sexual practices should always be used to reduce the chances of sexually transmitted infections, which should reduce the chance of re-activating Reiter's syndrome or of getting the problem in the first place. It is unlikely that much can be done to prevent Reiter's syndrome following gut infections as there is no way of telling in advance which people are susceptible. The only practical steps are to ensure good food hygiene and never eat undercooked meat or poultry (the commonest source of food poisoning). People who have suffered from Reiter's syndrome and are HLA-B27 positive are more likely to have further attacks if again exposed to similar infection.

Psoriatic arthritis

Psoriasis is a skin condition that affects about 2 per cent of the population. Usually it causes red scaly patches to appear on the skin and scalp and often there are changes in the fingernails in the form of tiny pits on the surface. About 5 per cent of people with psoriasis also develop an inflammatory arthritis. Rarely the arthritis precedes the skin changes, but usually psoriatic arthritis develops in someone who has had skin psoriasis for a while. The cause of psoriasis is unknown but about a third of people have a family history of it.

The pattern of joint inflammation associated with psoriasis is fairly characteristic. Most typical is inflammation of the small joints of the fingers next to the nails (DIP joints). Often the nails with the most surface pitting are those of the fingers with the most inflamed joints. Inflammation of the equivalent joint in the feet is also seen. As with all these types of arthritis there are common features, so there may be spinal arthritis or involvement of the limb joints.

Diagnosing psoriatic arthritis is not usually very difficult because of the pattern and the fact that the skin rash is usually present; however, it is important for the doctor not to assume too quickly that the two are related. It is possible, for example, for someone to have psoriasis as well as unrelated osteoarthritis affecting the DIP joints. X-rays of the hands (and feet if involved) usually show features that positively identify psoriatic arthritis.

Treatment is similar to AS and Reiter's syndrome. Sulfasalazine and methotrexate are the most commonly used DMARDs whereas the antimalarial drugs (chloroquine and hydroxychloroquine) are avoided as they can potentially cause the skin psoriasis to flare up. Steroids have to be used with caution in psoriasis for the same reason.

Key Points

- Ankylosing spondylitis, Reiter's syndrome and psoriatic arthritis are the main inflammatory joint diseases other than rheumatoid arthritis.
- These conditions have some similarities between each other, including involvement of the spine and the absence of rheumatoid factor in the blood.
- Treatment is along similar lines to that for rheumatoid arthritis.
- Sulfasalazine and methotrexate are the commonest DMARDs used for them, with the newer biological treatments such as Etanercept and Infliximab under trial.

Chapter 9

Connective Tissue Diseases

Connective tissue is the background support structure of the body. Like the steel frame inside a skyscraper it isn't visible from the outside – instead it surrounds and holds virtually every tissue and organ and acts like a packing material between all of the parts, including at the microscopic level. Connective tissue takes various physical forms depending on its exact site in the body, and according to the proportions of collagen and other substances it contains. Mixed throughout connective tissues are many of the cells of the immune system, and the connective tissue diseases are therefore those conditions that occur from activation of inflammation within connective tissues. Because they are so widely spread throughout the body connective tissue diseases can have a very wide range of symptoms and effects, and affect almost any organ or tissue. Arthritis is one of the main consequences, which is why connective tissue diseases appear in this book. There are many types of connective tissue disease but in each it appears that the affected person's immune system has become active in attacking their own tissues. Therefore they are also often referred to as the 'autoimmune diseases'. Rheumatoid arthritis is the main one and systemic lupus erythematosus (SLE) the best known of the remainder.

As with all such conditions the causes of them are really not understood. A combination of a genetic tendency to the condition, which is then triggered by some other factor, is probably correct but not very explicit.

Systemic lupus erythematosus (lupus)

SLE is a rare condition, present in about 30 people per 100,000 of the population. It is nine times more common in women compared with men, and nine times more common in the Afro-Caribbean population compared with white Caucasians. Most people with SLE are at or below middle age.

FEATURES AND COMPLICATIONS

SLE can affect a very wide range of tissues, so the pattern of the illness can vary a lot between individuals. General symptoms such as fatigue, weight loss and fever are common, as are joint pains, which usually involve many joints at a time.

Skin rashes appear in the majority of people with SLE. A red flush across the cheeks, called a butterfly rash, is particularly characteristic but other rashes over the body are common, and many are made worse by exposure to sunlight.

People with SLE have a much higher likelihood of developing hardening of the arteries (atherosclerosis) – the process that results in thickening and narrowing of the blood vessels. Atherosclerosis reduces the blood flowing through affected arteries, and the consequences of that depend on which organ is involved. In the brain, atherosclerosis may lead to a stroke, whereas in the heart, a heart attack can result.

Half of people with SLE develop inflammation of the membrane that covers the lungs, which leads to chest pain and sometimes breathlessness due to the build-up of fluid between the lungs and the inside of the rib cage. Inflammation of lung tissue may cause more significant breathlessness.

In as many as a third of people with SLE the kidneys can be significantly affected, causing damage to the filtering system and reducing the kidneys' ability to 'clean' the blood in the normal way. Careful monitoring of kidney function is required when there is evidence of damage, which can be detected with simple urine tests looking for excess protein or for red or white blood cells that have leaked into the urine.

Involvement of the brain and nervous system can take many forms. Mood disturbance or confusion, headaches and fits as well as a number of nerve problems are all possibilities.

This is not a complete list of the problems that are known to be potentially associated with SLE so it will be clear how wide-ranging these problems can be. Making a diagnosis may, however, be quite difficult in early SLE as fewer features will be present. Blood tests are often helpful in detecting or confirming SLE.

BLOOD TESTS

Anti-nuclear antibody (ANA) is positive in over 95 per cent of people with SLE and anti-DNA antibody is more or less specific for SLE if detected. Other tests such as the ESR and C-reactive protein level are likely to be raised, indicating there is activity of the immune system (chapter 4). A fairly common pattern in SLE is that the ESR is high but the C-reactive protein is normal but goes up if there is an infection somewhere or a sudden flare-up of the arthritis. Several other antibody tests are used by rheumatology specialists to help classify sub-types of SLE. Very high levels of anti-DNA antibody can be associated with a greater likelihood of kidney involvement from SLE.

TREATMENT OF SLE

General actions include using sunscreen creams and avoiding sun exposure when people have light-sensitive skin. It is very important that the risk of developing atherosclerosis is minimised, so the other factors that contribute to atherosclerosis (smoking, high blood pressure, high cholesterol) need to be checked and properly controlled. Every effort should be made to stop smoking.

A low fat diet with a high intake of oily fish may be of benefit in SLE, and can also be helpful in slowing the development of athero-sclerosis.

Drug therapy is complex and tailored to the individual. NSAIDs and other painkillers might be all that is needed when someone has early SLE and no evidence of other problems. Conversely someone with active SLE causing kidney damage will probably need high-dose steroid treatment and other drugs such as cyclophosphamide to dampen the immune system.

Steroids dampen SLE but in the long term they give rise to many side effects, as was noted in rheumatoid arthritis. Osteoporosis is more common in SLE and can be made worse by steroid treatment, so measures to protect bone strength are usually required. Of the 'DMARD' group of drugs used in RA, methotrexate and the antimalarial drug hydroxychloroquine are the main ones used in SLE. Combinations of the different drugs can be required, and the treatment of SLE requires a good deal of specialist expertise to achieve symptom control with the minimum of ill effects from the drugs.

SLE is a long-term illness, and like the other auto-immune diseases is controllable but not curable. People with it can get a lot of help and support not just from their specialist and primary care team but also from national and local support groups (appendix C).

Antiphospholipid syndrome (Hughes' syndrome)

Phospholipids are complex molecules of fat combined with phosphorus that are found widely throughout the body, particularly as components of the membranes that surround cells. The antiphospholipid syndrome

(APS) is a condition in which antibodies to these phospholipids are found and which is also associated with an increased tendency of the blood to clot, hence the term 'sticky blood syndrome'. Antiphospholipid syndrome can occur on its own, or in association with a connective tissue disease – which is usually SLE. Both types are more common in women.

The consequences of the blood clots caused by APS depend on where they are sited. In a leg vein for example this might lead to a deep vein thrombosis that could move up into the lung with possibly fatal consequences. In the arteries supplying the brain a stroke, or series of strokes, could result. In pregnancy small clots can occur within the placenta – the junction between the baby's and the mother's circulations – which raises the chance of miscarriage, particularly in mid-pregnancy. APS is a relatively newly discovered condition, first described in 1983 by Dr Graham Hughes, now Head of the Lupus Unit at St Thomas's Hospital in London. It is important to recognise it as treatment with 'blood-thinning' drugs (anticoagulants) reduces the likelihood of serious clots occurring.

DIAGNOSIS OF APS

A history of previous clotting problems such as deep vein thrombosis, stroke or heart attack, especially if occurring at a young age, should prompt a search for antiphospholipid antibodies in the blood. Less specific clues include headaches, migraine, memory loss and confusion although APS will only rarely be the cause of those symptoms.

TREATMENT OF ANTIPHOSPHOLIPID SYNDROME

Warfarin is the oral anticoagulant now commonly used for APS. An injectable anticoagulant called heparin is suitable for use in pregnant women with APS and may reduce the tendency to miscarriage. Some people are noted to have a positive antiphospholipid antibody test, but have never had a thrombosis or a miscarriage. Research into the best treatment for such patients is currently being carried out, but at present the recommended treatment is low dose aspirin. Aspirin acts on platelets (the small blood particles involved in forming clots) to reduce their stickiness, and hence reduces the ability of the blood to clot.

Polymyalgia rheumatica

'Polymyalgia' literally means 'pain from many muscles', which is a fair way to summarise this fairly common condition that affects middle aged to elderly adults. It is an auto-immune condition in which the tissues under attack are the linings of the arteries throughout the body. About one in 2000 people over 50 and as many as one in 100 over 70 have polymyalgia rheumatica (PMR). It is most common in Northern Europeans and unusual in Asian and black populations.

SYMPTOMS OF PMR

PMR causes pain and morning stiffness mainly in and around the shoulders and thighs (it may also affect the neck and torso). Sometimes it comes on quite abruptly but it is commoner for it to develop over several weeks or months. Often, a person with PMR cannot get out of bed without help and has difficulty climbing stairs. Prolonged rest or inactivity may increase the stiffness and activities such as driving become more difficult.

Other common complaints include feeling generally unwell, fatigue and depression. Occasionally, a slight fever accompanies the condition. Some people notice a loss of appetite and weight.

In about 15 per cent of people with PMR a painful inflammation occurs in the arteries in the head, particularly around the temple area: this is called 'temporal', or 'giant cell' arteritis. Temporal arteritis is particularly important to diagnose as without treatment it can lead to blindness. Fuller details follow below.

Unlike SLE, polymyalgia rheumatica does not have any tendency to damage other tissues such as the liver, kidney or lung.

DIAGNOSING PMR

The two most useful blood tests are the erythrocyte sedimentation rate (ESR) and/or the C-reactive protein (CRP) test (chapter 4). Both of these tests give a broad indication that there is some inflammatory process going on somewhere in the body and classically in PMR the readings are very high (for example the ESR is usually over 50 mm per hour). Other tests are done to rule out conditions that can look like PMR, such as rheumatoid arthritis or fibromyalgia (a painful muscle syndrome accompanied by fatigue). There is no specific test for PMR and the main point a doctor needs to bear in mind is the possibility of the diagnosis in the first place. It can be the case that aches and pains, and even depression, are just put down wrongly to 'old age'. As PMR is highly treatable, missing the diagnosis does the patient a considerable disservice.

TREATMENT

Corticosteroid drugs are the mainstay of treatment and improvement is often very rapid (within 24–48 hours). Injectable forms of corticosteroid can be used if preferred although they do not give any better results and need to be repeated every three weeks or so. Unfortunately steroids need to be given for at least two and often as many as six years in the majority of people with PMR and withdrawn very slowly to avoid relapse. There can therefore be problems with long-term steroid side effects but fortunately most people with PMR can be kept well with a small dose of steroid, so the risk of side effects is fairly low. Bone protection is required for people on long-term steroids to reduce the likelihood of developing osteoporosis.

Where there is difficulty getting the dose low enough (below about 10mg of prednisolone daily) then other drugs (DMARDs) can be added that dampen the immune system. These may allow the steroid dose to be dropped a bit although the evidence that they are effective in PMR is not strong either way.

Giant cell arteritis (temporal arteritis, cranial arteritis)

This can be considered the 'severe version of PMR' although it is probably a separate condition with many features in common. The main symptom is sudden onset throbbing headache in one or both temples. The pain can also be felt elsewhere, such as at the back of the head or be just a generalised headache. It can be severe enough to keep someone awake. The inflamed artery might be tender to touch as it runs under the skin of the temple, although this is not a very reliable finding.

GCA is uncommon in people under 50 years old, but if these symptoms arise in an older person then the diagnosis really needs to be confirmed very quickly. The inflammation present in the arteries of the temple is also present in other arteries of the head, notably those taking blood to the eyes, and inflamed arteries are at risk of becoming blocked. In the eye this could cause permanent blindness. Fortunately GCA responds quickly to corticosteroids and if treated before any visual loss occurs the threat to sight will be removed. The gold standard test for diagnosing GCA is to take a tissue sample (biopsy) from the artery itself. Under the microscope this will reveal the presence of the 'giant' inflammatory cells that give the condition its name. As steroid drugs reverse these changes quickly the biopsy needs to be done before starting them or very soon afterwards (within a few days at the most). However, it is not always possible to get a quick biopsy for logistic reasons, so often the diagnosis is based on the patient's history, along with the blood test results, so that treatment can be started promptly.

As in polymyalgia rheumatica, steroids should be given for at least two to three years in giant cell arteritis. Having a biopsy-confirmed diagnosis at the start makes it much easier to justify committing to this length of treatment but the risk to eyesight of untreated GCA is high, so it is safer to act on the grounds of a strong clinical diagnosis if a biopsy cannot be obtained.

Key Points

- The connective tissue diseases are auto-immune conditions involving the basic support tissues throughout the body.
- Systemic lupus erythematosus (SLE) is the main example and is much commoner in women and in people of Afro-Caribbean origin.
- SLE can potentially affect joints, skin, heart, lungs and kidneys but can generally be controlled with steroid and other anti-inflammatory drugs.
- Antiphospholipid syndrome (Hughes' syndrome) is a blood-clotting problem that can accompany SLE or occur on its own. It is treated with long-term anticoagulant (blood-thinning) drugs.
- Polymyalgia rheumatica (PMR) is an inflammatory condition of arteries that affects older adults and shows as marked morning stiffness of the muscles. It responds well to steroids.
- Giant cell arteritis is similar to PMR and is potentially sight threatening. It also responds well to steroids.

Chapter 10

Gout and Pseudogout

Whereas rheumatoid arthritis is the most common inflammatory arthritis in women over 40, for men it is gout that takes the lead – affecting six per thousand adult males. Gout is eight times commoner in men than women. In gout there is inflammation of affected joints as well as of tendons and soft tissues. Lumps under the skin can appear and gout sufferers are at risk of kidney stones and, rarely, kidney damage.

The underlying problem in gout relates to the body's production of a natural substance called uric acid. Uric acid is the end product of metabolism in the body of a type of protein called purine and normally it is eliminated through the urine (mostly) and the faeces. In people with a predisposition to gout, uric acid accumulates in the blood. Among some of these people the concentration in the blood is so high that the uric acid 'overflows' and settles in the joints and possibly in the skin.

Types of gout

The are two kinds of gout:

1 PRIMARY

This is due to a genetic tendency for uric acid elimination to be naturally slow, so even in normal circumstances it tends to build up in the blood. Having a naturally high level of uric acid in the blood is called 'primary hyperuricaemia'. Prior to the onset of symptoms of gout, there is usually a latent period of several years in which the concentration of uric acid in the blood has gradually increased. This condition is called 'asymptomatic hyperuricaemia'; however, it's important to note that 95 per cent of people with a raised uric acid level never develop gout.

2 SECONDARY

Here the gout is caused by another disease that produces uric acid faster than the body can eliminate it. An example is following anti-cancer therapy where the treatment causes the destruction of large numbers of cancerous cells and as a result there is a sudden release of uric acid. Alternatively, secondary gout occurs as a side effect of a drug that causes the elimination of uric acid to be impaired. Some diuretics (water pills) are prone to doing this, as is aspirin.

Symptoms

A first attack of gout typically occurs in a man around 40 to 60 years old, often at night and the favoured joint is the base of the big toe (the first metatarsal joint, or 1st MTP, if you remember your terms from chapter 4!). Such pain from the foot is called 'podagra', which is an old alternative term for gout. If it is the knee that is sore it is called 'gonagra'. Usually gout attacks one joint at a time and quite why the first MTP gets picked out so often is unclear. It probably relates to the mechanical stress that occurs in this joint in walking, which in some way encourages uric acid crystals to form in the joint. Under the microscope uric acid crystals are long and needle-shaped and it is not difficult to imagine why they can trigger an inflammatory reaction. An affected big toe looks red or shiny purple, swollen and angry and it can be too painful to support the weight of a bed sheet, let alone walk on it.

The first attack usually subsides after about a week. About 10 per cent of people will never again experience gout and about 60 per cent will have a similar or more severe attack within the next year. Some will go on having repeated attacks, which can produce permanent joint damage. If no preventive treatment is undertaken then, over time, uric acid mixed with inflammatory cells and scar tissue accumulates under the skin. This shows as small bumps called tophi near the joints or on the outer side of the ear. Occasionally these rupture and ooze yellowish chalky material. Gout can affect any of the main joints such as the knees and ankles, elbows, wrists and hands but curiously it tends to skip the spine, hips and shoulders.

Diagnosis

Ideally gout is confirmed by finding uric acid crystals in the synovial fluid taken from an affected joint. If this is not possible then X-rays of joints that have suffered repeated attacks of gout may confirm the diagnosis but this will not work for joints that have not yet been damaged. The blood level of uric acid is usually, but not always, raised during an acute attack of gout and in any case many people have high uric acid levels and never get gout – so there can be times when the diagnosis is unclear. Once a couple of attacks have occurred it becomes much easier to see that the pattern fits with gout.

Treatment and prevention

Rest of the inflamed joint combined with a non-steroidal anti-inflammatory drug (usually given at a high dosage for the first few days) are the initial steps. A good fluid intake will help flush out uric acid from the kidneys. Aspirin should be avoided as a painkiller as it holds back uric acid from being released by the kidney, and so can make the attack worse. An old drug called colchicine is still in use for acute attacks but it often causes digestive upset and is not first choice. If someone cannot take a NSAID (see chapter 6) then it is feasible sometimes for a specialist to inject steroids into a joint. Oral steroids can also be used but often the people who cannot take a NSAID are the same ones who cannot take oral steroids, perhaps because of a history of stomach bleeding for example. Exoricoxib is a CoX-2 selective NSAID that has been shown to be as effective as the most powerful commonly used NSAID (indometacin) for gout, but has fewers side effects.

Prevention of further attacks of gout in the long term depends on lowering the level of uric acid, and this is most effectively done with an oral drug called allopurinol. Allopurinol blocks one of the enzymes involved in the production of uric acid, thus lowering the blood level. It needs to be started a couple of weeks after an acute attack of gout has settled and initially at a low dose which is then built up to the full dose over a month or so. Starting it too soon or at too high an initial dose can itself trigger another attack. Continuing a NSAID during the first month also helps reduce the chance of a flare-up. Allopurinol is a well-tolerated drug but occasionally can cause skin rashes. Someone who is found to have a raised uric acid level (asymptomatic hyperuricaemia) but who has no family history of gout and no history of a gout attack does not need to take drugs to lower the uric acid level.

Gout and heart disease

For reasons that are not well understood, people who get gout are also more likely to have high blood pressure and coronary heart disease (hardening of the arteries of the heart). They are also more likely to be overweight and perhaps to have diabetes. An attack of gout should therefore also be taken as a signal to the doctor to check the person's blood pressure, cholesterol, weight and smoking history and advise changes as necessary. Having asymptomatic hyperuricaemia alone probably does not increase the risk of developing circulatory disease.

Pseudogout

This is a type of arthritis that is also due to crystals appearing in the joint, but of a different material called calcium pyrophosphate. When sufficient calcium pyrophosphate builds up in the cartilage of a joint it shows up on X-rays as a thin line but, as with gout, diagnosis is really only confirmed if crystals of the substance are found in the synovial fluid taken from an inflamed joint.

What causes the build-up of the crystals is unknown but a number of conditions are associated with pseudogout including under-activity of the thyroid gland (which controls the body's overall metabolism), overactivity of the parathyroid glands (which control the amount of calcium in the blood) and a disorder called haemo-chromatosis which leads to excess iron being absorbed and stored in the body.

The patterns of arthritis attacks caused by pseudogout are similar to those of gout except that the joints usually involved are the knee, wrist or shoulder. Pseudogout responds to painkillers such as NSAIDs but there is no equivalent treatment to prevent recurrence of attacks in the same way that allopurinol protects against recurrent attacks of gout. Making a diagnosis of pseudogout can be quite difficult as the arthritis attacks are not usually as dramatic or quite as painful as gout and the crystals of calcium pyrophosphate can be hard to find in synovial fluid samples. Special laboratories around the country can help in this regard.

There are other rare forms of arthritis due to different types of crystal but their management follows the same lines as those above.

Key Points

- Gout is the commonest inflammatory arthritis in older men.
- It is due to excess uric acid appearing in the joints.
- Secondary causes of gout include the use of diuretic drugs.

- A raised level of uric acid in the blood in the absence of other factors such as a family or personal history of gout does not need to be treated.
- Allopurinol is a drug used long term to protect against repeated attacks of gout.
- Gout can be associated with other risk factors for heart and circulatory disease.
- Other forms of crystal-related arthritis exist, such as pseudo-gout due to calcium pyrophosphate. They are treated in similar ways to gout but protective drug therapy is not available for them.

Chapter 11

Osteoporosis

Osteoporosis is the condition in which the amount of bone tissue in the body is reduced below what is normal for a person, taking into account their sex and age. Put simply, osteoporosis causes weaker bones, and thus increases the likelihood of breaking a bone. Strictly speaking it is not a disease of joints and so arguably it should not occupy a chapter in a book about arthritis! Osteoporosis is, however, a very important bone condition that is often misunderstood or neglected. This more than justifies its inclusion here.

Bone structure

Bone really is quite astonishing stuff. It has a complex structure that achieves the maximum amount of strength for the least amount of weight, it can increase its thickness in areas subjected to repeated heavy loads, repair itself when broken and as a sideline is the site of manufacture of most of the components of blood (the bone marrow).

If one takes a typical bone such as the femur (upper leg bone) and cuts it across one sees there is an outer shell of very hard bone while in the middle space it has a honeycomb structure, through which is mingled the bone marrow. Bone is made up mostly of collagen fibres upon which are laid down crystals made from calcium and phosphate that give bone its ability to withstand compression and bending forces. It is possible to take a bone and chemically leach these minerals out – bone that has been thus treated becomes quite flexible and rubbery.

If one looks at bone under the microscope one sees that scattered throughout are two types of specialised cells. One type continually makes new bone (these are called 'osteoblasts') and the other group continuously dissolves bone into its component materials (the 'osteoclasts'). Bone is therefore not a static or inert tissue – it is always on the go and the actions of bone manufacture and disassembly are usually exactly balanced. When increased loads are repeatedly put upon a bone then the osteoblasts become a little bit more active, thus laying down more bone locally and increasing the strength of this region. When a bone is fractured, osteoblasts go into overdrive around the fracture site and lay down more collagen fibres, then minerals on top to strengthen them. In osteoporosis the opposite happens and, usually over years, the osteoclasts dissolve a bit more bone than is replaced, thus one ends up with weaker bones (figure 4). Fractures in bone affected by osteoporosis are most likely in areas where there is a greater percentage of the honeycomb type of bone, which is less able to take the shock of a fall. These are the wrist, the femur close to the hip joint (called the 'neck' of the femur) and the vertebrae of the lower spine.

The scale of the problem

One in three women and one in 12 men over the age of 50 will suffer a fracture of the hip, wrist or spine as a result of osteoporosis, which in total causes 310,000 fractures in the UK annually. Hip and wrist fractures usually result from falls, whereas fractures of the spine tend

Figure 4: Normal and osteoporotic bone structures

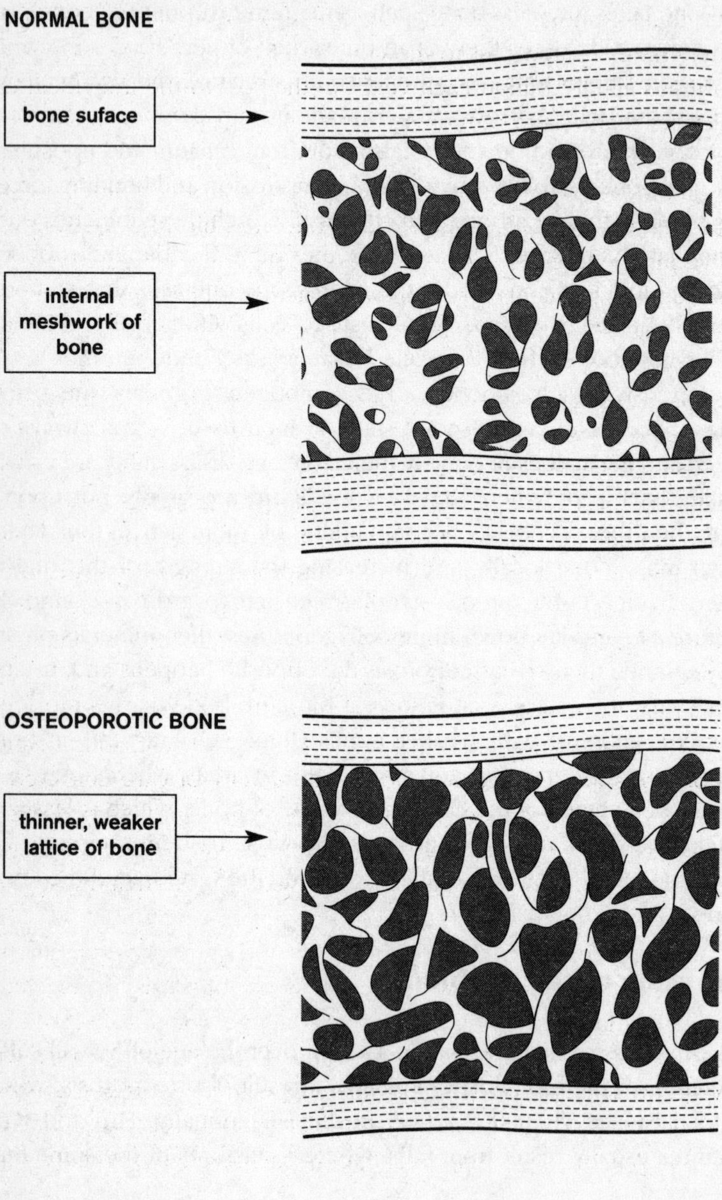

NORMAL BONE

bone suface →

internal meshwork of bone →

OSTEOPOROTIC BONE

thinner, weaker lattice of bone →

to occur spontaneously when a vertebra that has been weakening for some time crumples under the stress of supporting the weight of the body. The estimated cost to the country of treating these fractures is enormous at £1.7 billion each year but the cost to the individual can be higher than a sum of money:

- Bone fractures can cause considerable pain and disability.
- 50 per cent of people who suffer a fractured hip lose the ability to live independently.
- Around 20 per cent of people who fracture a hip die within a year as a result of their fracture.

The majority of people who suffer a fracture from osteoporosis are however not known to have the condition prior to breaking their bone. Osteoporosis is an under-recognised condition, which is partly because in the UK we have not developed an organised approach to detecting it. As a result we do not yet consistently seek people at high risk of getting a fracture and offer them appropriate advice or treatment to reduce their risk. Many people who have had a fracture due to osteoporosis do not receive follow-up treatment that helps reduce the chance of their getting another one.

There are very wide variations between the different regions of the UK in the quality and quantity of effort put in to detecting and treating osteoporosis and further divisions in the quality of care delivered to people from different social groups. In a recent study carried out in Glasgow, people from the most deprived areas were eight times less likely to be referred for the tests to detect osteoporosis than those from the most affluent areas.

There is, however, some good news too. The government has recognised the deficiencies that exist in osteoporosis management nationally and more funding is slowly coming through to expand the services, such as bone scanning machines to help diagnose it as well as specialists in osteoporosis. A 'Primary Care Strategy for Osteoporosis and Falls' has just been published (October 2002) that sets out standards for osteoporosis care that ought to be achieved by Primary Care

Organisations (see appendix C). As with all such initiatives the publication of a document, although important, won't achieve much without the other resources coming along to match.

In fairness it has to be said that as yet osteoporosis is not fully understood. Although we know much about what increases the risk of a person getting it, we know of only some things that can be done to prevent osteoporosis. As we'll see though, you can do many things to help yourself, as part of a healthy approach to life. Being better informed about osteoporosis will enable you to help yourself but will also help you to ask the right questions if you need more information about or treatment for the condition.

Definitions

It is normal for bone to get a bit weaker each year after the age of about 30, when our bones are at their maximum strength. Men tend to have greater bone mass than women of the same age. For a few years after the menopause women experience an increased rate of bone loss, which is secondary to the drop in oestrogen that is part of the hormone change occurring during the menopause (oestrogen has a protective effect upon bone strength). Defining when bones are abnormally weak therefore has to take account of what is normal for the two sexes and the different age groups and so to some extent is a mathematical exercise. Modern bone scanning devices can measure the density of bones and have allowed doctors to build up a range of readings across large numbers of people that set the range for normal bone strength. Osteoporosis can therefore be said to be present if a person's bone density measurement is significantly low compared to these standards.

A person is also deemed to have osteoporosis if they have suffered a fracture too easily, i.e. a 'low impact' or 'osteoporotic' fracture. This is something of a circular definition but nonetheless identifying people who have osteoporosis after they have suffered the consequences and concentrating upon them efforts at prevention reduces the chance of their suffering another fracture later. A low trauma fracture is one that occurs from a fall from standing height or less and fractures of the hip, wrist or forearm can be categorised in this way fairly easily. It is more difficult to do so for the spine as many spinal fractures occur out of the blue and are not related to falls – sometimes they are not even accompanied by much pain. However, the sudden onset of back pain should suggest there has been a collapsed vertebra, possibly due to osteoporosis.

Causes of osteoporosis

Various factors are known to increase the rate at which bone loss occurs, and they can be divided into three groups:

1 those that one can do nothing about,
2 those that are under one's own control,
3 causes related to other medical conditions or drug therapy.

1 UNCHANGEABLE CAUSES OF INCREASED BONE LOSS
- Increasing age
- Family history of osteoporosis
- Female sex
- Following natural menopause
- Being thin (see below)

2 CHANGEABLE CAUSES OF INCREASED BONE LOSS
- Inactivity
- Poor diet (low in calcium)
- Smoking
- Increased alcohol intake

3 MEDICALLY-RELATED CAUSES OF INCREASED BONE LOSS

- Steroid drug treatment (especially if prolonged more than a few weeks).
- Early menopause or the removal of the ovaries at a young age (under 45 years).
- Hormone abnormalities (such as over-activity of the thyroid gland, or of the glands which produce the body's natural steroids, or under-production of testosterone in men).

These are the main, but not all the possible, conditions that can lead to osteoporosis.

Diagnosing osteoporosis

The best test to diagnose osteoporosis is a scan to determine the density of the bones. Usually the same reference point in the skeleton is chosen, which allows better comparison between different people. The hip, forearm, heel bone or spine can all be used but exactly which varies according to local procedure. Although there are several technical ways in which a bone scan can be done the best is currently the 'DEXA' scan – short for dual-energy X-ray absorpiometry. As the name implies, a DEXA scan uses X-rays to determine the density of bone. Ultrasound of the heel bone is another common technique and uses cheaper equipment but it is not yet clear if it is as accurate or reliable as DEXA scanning.

Ordinary X-rays are not reliable as a tool for diagnosing osteoporosis, for various technical reasons. It can be possible to suspect from a standard X-ray film that the person has less bone mass than normal as the bone outline on the film might appear fainter, but the same appearance will show if the exposure of the film is slightly too high. Conversely if the film is slightly underexposed then the bones will look normally dense. In any case as much as 30 per cent of bone mass needs to be lost before it shows up on ordinary X-rays. DEXA scanning is designed to get round these limitations.

One of the problems in the UK is that there are not yet enough of these DEXA scanners to make the test freely available, so some form of vetting procedure is used to ensure that those most at need of being scanned are tested. The details of these criteria vary a bit around the country but could look like this list, in which the presence of any one factor would justify a DEXA scan:

- A woman over 50 who has had a low trauma fracture.
- Anyone taking oral steroid (prednisolone 5mg daily or greater for three or more months).
- A woman under 45 who has had an early menopause or removal of the ovaries.
- A woman who is around the menopause who also has any two of the following:

1 Smokes
2 Has a body mass index (BMI – see below) less than 21
3 Has a history in her mother of a hip fracture below 80 years of age
4 Drinks more than 35 units of alcohol weekly (see below).

- A man with a high alcohol consumption, of over 50 units of alcohol weekly.

People who are unusually thin are more likely to develop osteoporosis, and the way to define 'thin-ness' is to measure the body mass index (BMI). The BMI relates a person's weight to their height and therefore can be applied to any person, whether tall or short, and to both sexes.

BODY MASS INDEX

Weight and height are related and knowledge of both is needed before one can say if a person is overweight, underweight or just right. A simple mathematical formula relating the two is now universally used to do this – the Body Mass Index (BMI). To calculate a BMI, take the person's weight (in kilograms) and divide it by the square of their height (in metres). For example an 80kg person of height 1.7m will have a BMI of 80/(1.7x1.7)= 27.7 kg/m^2 (the BMI formula applies equally to men and women). The ranges of BMI are:

- Normal   = 20–24.9
- Overweight   = 25–30
- Obese   = Over 30

People with a BMI of 21 or less have a higher rate of bone loss than those who are heavier, and obese people have lower rates of bone loss than those who are ideal weight. It is not known if a thin person who deliberately puts on a lot of weight will reduce their subsequent fracture risk. Obesity of course carries with it many other health hazards.

ALCOHOL

Historically the recommended maximum consumption of alcohol per week is 21 units for women and 28 units for men. High levels of alcohol intake (over 50 units per week in men, or 35 units in women) are definitely associated with osteoporosis, as well as all the other serious health risks that accompany alcoholism. It is possible that lower levels of alcohol consumption than this could still damage bone as well as be associated with other health problems such as raised blood pressure or diabetes. Many experts therefore now recommend lower safe limits of alcohol consumption of 21 units weekly for men and 14 units weekly for women.

A unit of alcohol is:

- 250ml (½ pint) of ordinary strength beer/lager
- 1 glass (125ml/4 fl oz) of wine
- 1 pub measure of sherry/vermouth (1.5oz)
- 1 pub measure of spirits (1.5oz)

Prevention and treatment

GENERAL MEASURES

Osteoporosis is ideally a condition that should be prevented from occurring, but that is an unrealistic aim given our present state of knowledge and ability to influence it. It should, however, be obvious from the above that healthy bones at least partially reflect healthy living. Taking regular exercise is the single most important action anyone can take to improve the strength of their bones. Exercise also greatly reduces the risk of heart disease, high blood pressure and diabetes and it has positive effects on mental well-being too. The sort of exercise that is beneficial is weight bearing, such as walking or aerobics. Excessive running may however cause increased bone loss and as some running enthusiasts are also very thin they should take advice on the best way to avoid bone problems later in life. The majority of us who are not in the elite athlete category need not be so concerned.

Stopping smoking should be a priority for anyone interested in enjoying a longer life as well as keeping away from orthopaedic wards, and alcohol consumption should be kept within safe limits.

DIET

A good calcium intake is essential throughout life for healthy bones and there is good evidence that the adequacy of a child's diet at least partially determines their osteoporosis risk in adulthood. Although dairy products are high in calcium they are not the only source. Non-dairy food sources include:

- nuts and pulses (almonds, Brazil nuts, hazelnuts, sesame seeds),
- green leafy vegetables (broccoli, spinach, watercress, curly kale),
- dried fruits (apricots, dates, figs),
- fish (mackerel, pilchards, salmon, sardines),
- tofu and various calcium-fortified foods.

The daily intake of calcium required by an adult is around 800 milligrams. On average 250ml or half a pint of cow's milk or 150g/5oz of yoghurt contains 300 milligrams of calcium and low-fat dairy products contain the same amount of calcium as higher fat varieties. Calcium supplements can be bought and there are several types available on prescription if someone's dietary intake is low or marginal. Frail, elderly people with poor mobility may be helped by taking a supplement of calcium along with vitamin D. This type of supplement is safe but is best discussed with a doctor first.

These general measures can be used by everyone, whether or not they ultimately are shown to have osteoporosis. More detailed intervention depends on individual circumstances and so only an overview can be presented here. There are several types of treatment available, and often a combination will be more appropriate than just one.

HORMONE REPLACEMENT THERAPY

Oestrogen seems to protect bone strength and the drop in oestrogen that occurs following the menopause is mirrored by an increased loss of bone for a few years thereafter. The loss continues but less steeply in older women. Hormone replacement therapy replaces oestrogen and so reduces the rate of bone loss. The pros and cons of HRT are many, and are presently the subject of much debate. It may be several years yet before we have clearer ideas about which women would be best given HRT from the osteoporosis point of view but in general this would be the likely choice for a woman up to about the age of 55 who was at high risk of developing it.

SELECTIVE ESTROGEN RECEPTOR MODULATOR (SERM)

This is a fairly new type of drug, of which raloxifene (Evista) is presently the only available one. Raloxifene stimulates bone growth just as oestrogens do but has an anti-oestrogen effect on the uterus (womb) and on breast tissue. The latter effect is seen as desirable as it may reduce the tendency for long-term oestrogen-based HRT to increase the risk of developing breast cancer. Raloxifene may however increase the risk of developing blood clots in the veins and cannot be used by a woman with a past history of DVT. It is preferably used only in women who are five years past their menopause and would be an option for a woman between about 55 and 70 years of age. It has been shown to reduce the occurrence of spinal fractures, but not hip fractures.

BISPHOSPHONATES

This is a group of drugs that slows the rate at which bone is dissolved, thus favouring a build-up in bone strength over time. Two types are in common use: alendronate (Fosamax) and etidronate (Didronel PMO). There are slight differences between them in the available preparations and in how frequently they are taken but they act in the same way. Alendronate is described more fully in appendix B. Alendronate and etidronate can be used in men and women who have osteoporosis or are at risk of developing it, including where this is secondary to the use of steroid drugs. Risendronate is another bisphosphonate used only in women after the menopause but otherwise is similar to the others. Alendronate and risendronate reduce the occurrence of fractures of the hip and spine, whereas etidronate has been shown to do so only for the spine.

OTHER TREATMENTS

These are quite specialised and not commonly used. Calcitonin is a hormone given by injection but it is less effective than HRT or the bisphosphonates and has a number of potential side effects, including allergic reactions. Calcitriol is a vitamin D-like compound that can be used in osteoporosis caused by steroid drugs.

Hip protectors are shock-absorbing pads that can be worn to cushion the impact over the hip bone should a person fall down. They spread the load across a wider area of the upper leg and are useful as an extra measure in an elderly person prone to falls. They come as a sort of girdle with padding at the sides but some people may not always remember to put it on, or wish to keep it on.

Compliance is the business of sticking to the prescribed treatment, whether it is tablets or protective clothing and as osteoporosis treatment and prevention needs to be taken for years poor compliance can be a major issue in treating the condition. Elderly people are the most at risk of falls, and are also the most likely to become muddled about pills or suffer more severe side effects from them. Those in sheltered or supervised environments can be given help to remember their medication but where this is not possible and someone is forgetful then using a once weekly dose form of bisphosphonate supervised by a carer or nurse might be more reliable than a daily dose that depended entirely on the patient.

Osteoporosis and men

Women tend to get more coverage in osteoporosis than men as they live longer, have generally weaker bones and ultimately form the majority of people who have an osteoporotic fracture. Men do, however, also develop osteoporosis and show an increase in osteoporotic hip fractures after the age of about 70 similar to that shown by women five to 10 years younger. Men do not of course experience the recognisable hormone shift represented by the menopause in women, but they do experience a steady drop in output of testosterone (the 'male hormone') by the testes as they get older. Like oestrogen in women, testosterone has a protective effect on bone.

A very low level of testosterone can be suspected if there are obvious physical signs such as an absence of beard growth in a man but other, more subtle symptoms are also thought to be possibly due to testosterone lack. These include depression, nervousness, fatigue, poor concentration and memory, flushes and sweats, decreased libido and difficulty obtaining a satisfactory erection. This is a controversial area and experts remain uncertain how definite is this phenomenon of the 'male menopause'.

The situation is not helped by the fact that no easy test for this condition exists. Low blood levels of testosterone are insufficient to make the diagnosis because there is widespread disagreement over what is the normal range of testosterone levels and exactly what form of testosterone should be measured in the blood. The timing of the blood sample matters too, as testosterone is released into the bloodstream in pulses, and levels vary through the day.

Perhaps most important is being aware of the possibility of osteoporosis in a man who has had a fracture at a relatively young age, for example, or after relatively little trauma, or who shows signs of height loss or whose spine X-rays are suggestive of some bone loss. Very often the penny simply does not drop, yet men can also benefit from all of the general and more specific treatments, other than HRT, that apply to women. Testosterone treatment is controversial and uncertain in value in the majority of men who do not have very low testosterone levels so osteoporosis management should be along the lines of encouraging exercise and diet supplements as well as the other lifestyle measures, and bisphosphonate drugs when more active treatment is required.

Key Points

- Osteoporosis is the condition in which bone mass and strength are reduced from normal.
- Bone is an active tissue in which the processes of bone manufacture and removal are normally in balance.
- Bone strength naturally declines with age and is less in women than in men of the same age.
- The rate of bone loss increases for a few years in women following the menopause.
- Men also experience osteoporosis but have fewer fractures compared to women.
- Diagnosing osteoporosis is most accurately done by DEXA scans of bone density.

- Everyone can help to protect themselves against osteoporosis by adopting a healthy lifestyle and in particular by remaining as active as possible.
- Adequate dietary calcium intake should be ensured in everyone, if necessary with the addition of calcium supplements.
- The main specific treatments and preventive measures for osteoporosis include hormone replacement therapy and SERM treatment for women and bisphosphonate treatment for both sexes.
- People on long-term oral steroids should receive bone protection with bisphosphonates.

Chapter 12

Back Pain and Sciatica

The human spine is robust and flexible but it is also the source of much trouble. Pain in the lower back is one of the commonest reasons for someone to see a doctor and over 70 per cent of people in developed countries suffer low back pain at some point in their lives.

Many of the possible causes of spinal pain have been covered earlier in this book, such as osteoarthritis of the interlocking joints between vertebrae, involvement of the spine in several types of inflammatory arthritis and fractures of the vertebrae in spinal osteoporosis. Yet about 90 per cent of people who get back pain do not have any significant disease of the spine.

Ninety per cent of episodes of low back pain heal up within about six weeks but between 2 and 7 per cent of episodes go on to give long-term pain. About half of people who recover from an episode will have another one within the following two years. The effect of back pain on work absence is huge – up to three quarters of all absenteeism from work may be due to this cause alone.

Acute back pain means one of sudden onset, whereas chronic back pain refers to episodes that have gone on for several weeks or longer. Although they have a lot in common (you can't have chronic pain without first having acute pain), there are some differences in approach to the two problems.

Acute back pain

Sudden pain due to an excessively heavy lift is usually due to strain of muscles and ligaments rather than bony damage, but one has to remember the possibility of a spinal fracture, as mentioned in the previous chapter. Pain from either cause can be severe but painkillers such as paracetamol, aspirin, paracetamol/codeine combinations and NSAIDs are all likely to give some relief. Stronger painkillers are often needed for spinal fractures. It is part of the assessment of someone with such a problem to look for possible underlying causes, even if they are usually not found. Much depends on the symptoms and on the findings on examination but blood tests and X-rays looking for inflammatory conditions, signs of trauma or of bone disease may be required in the short term if the pain is particularly bad, if there is some delay in recovery or if there are any other features to raise the doctor's suspicions. Most of these tests can be organised by the GP.

Although a short spell of rest might be needed it is clear that in the vast majority of people with acute back pain bed rest of longer than a couple of days' duration does more harm than good. Prolonged rest lets people stiffen up and lose fitness, weakens muscles, emphasises the feeling of disability and actually amplifies the pain. People who keep active (with the help of painkillers if necessary) do better and are less likely to go on to have chronic pain. Specific back exercises, physiotherapy or other treatments like acupuncture have not been shown to have any definite benefit in acute back pain although an individual's experience may well be different. Some people who are prone to a pattern of recurrent back pain do find that a course of massage or treatment from a skilled physiotherapist, osteopath, chiropractor or similar therapist gives them quicker relief than waiting to get better on their own. The essential message though is to keep on the move.

An acute episode of back pain should prompt a look at how to stop it happening again if for example it has been the result of a work injury. Even if not so directly related it may be helpful to ensure that back care is given more attention in the future, so that one makes a habit of sitting comfortably at a desk or computer station, lifts objects with a straight back, avoids prolonged standing in a bent forward position, has adequate lumbar support in sofas and soft chairs and tries to avoid all the other ways we tend to abuse our backs without thinking, until a problem arises.

Sciatica

The sciatic nerves are two large bundles of nerve fibres that exit from the lower spine on each side and run down each leg, dividing into numerous other branches that eventually reach to the furthest points of the toes. Each nerve runs through the buttocks and then down the backs of the legs at first. The nerve is connected to the lower spinal cord, which is protected by the bony arches that project from the back of each vertebra (figure 5). Between each vertebra is the intervertebral disc – a cushion made of a tough but slightly flexible outer sheath surrounding a jelly-like core. The discs allow movement between each vertebra and take the shock loads of body weight and lifting etc. Weakening of the outer layers can allow the core to bulge, which in turn may cause pressure upon the nerve roots, which are immediately nearby. This is what really happens in a 'slipped disc'. Discs do not actually slip but they bulge and trap the nerves, which causes pain, numbness or lack of muscle power (or any combination thereof) in the region to which the squeezed nerve is connected. When this happens to the sciatic nerve roots the classic symptom of 'sciatica' develops, which is pain down the back of the leg, possibly reaching to the foot. Sciatica is an uncommon event compared to the total number

Figure 5a: Spinal cord and nerve roots in spinal cord

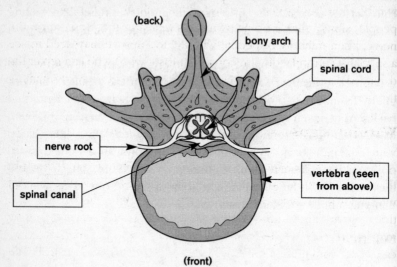

(back)

bony arch

spinal cord

nerve root

spinal canal

vertebra (seen from above)

(front)

Figure 5b: Prolapsed ('slipped') disc – a side view of the lower (lumbar) spine

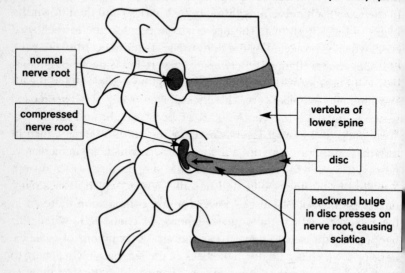

normal nerve root

compressed nerve root

vertebra of lower spine

disc

backward bulge in disc presses on nerve root, causing sciatica

of back pain episodes that occur but it usually means that recovery will be more prolonged. The disc bulge will, in the vast majority of people, slowly shrink on its own, thus relieving the pressure on the nerve, but a minority of people who fail to improve may need to see a specialist (orthopaedic surgeon or neurosurgeon) who can repair the damaged disc or remove the offending disc fragments that are jamming the nerves.

Warning signs

Although most episodes of acute back pain get better with little more than painkillers and the passage of time things can sometimes get worse. Of most importance is when the disc bulge gets bigger and threatens the nerves that control the bladder or the bowels. Surgery may then be needed urgently to relieve the pressure. Failure to do so can cause long-term problems with bladder or bowel control. The lowest part of the spinal cord is where these critical nerves arise and in appearance the spinal cord here looks like a horse's tail, with its numerous branches spreading out in a finely arranged bundle appropriately called the 'cauda equina'.

The 'cauda equina syndrome' (CES) is the name given to the urgent situation referred to above and it is not common. Because of its importance, however, it is worth knowing the symptoms (called 'red flag symptoms') that indicate it. The appearance of any red flag symptom should always be reported urgently to a doctor:

- Difficulty stopping or starting the stream of urine or controlling the bowel.
- Difficulty walking.
- Numbness in the 'saddle zone', i.e. the area between the legs that would be in contact with a bicycle saddle.

Chronic back pain

This is defined as pain that has not cleared up after 12 weeks but it is more complex than acute pain that has lasted a long time. Most people with chronic back pain do not have serious spinal disease and will not be any better off for seeing a specialist. Investigations looking for a physical cause for the pain are more than likely to turn up nothing abnormal, or to show coincidental findings that do not explain or relate adequately to the degree of pain being experienced.

Several factors appear to be important in predicting which people are likely to develop chronic back pain. For example, when the initial episode of pain is part of a wider problem of generalised pains or if it is accompanied by restriction of movement of the spine or by radiation of pain down the legs then it is more likely that chronic pain will result. People who smoke, who are unhappy at work, who report high levels of psychological stress or rate their own health as poor and who are relatively inactive are all more likely to suffer chronic pain.

People with chronic back pain are likely to report that painkillers, including NSAIDs, are only partially helpful. GPs can provide painkillers, advise on other types of therapy and on employment issues, detect the minority of people who might need to see a specialist and provide general support but they can't cure chronic back pain.

Understandably chronic back pain can sometimes lead to depression, and equally importantly depression can sometimes be the root cause of pain.

Most episodes of back pain are, fortunately, relatively short-lived and only a minority of people get long-term problems. Helping someone with chronic back pain requires far more than a mechanical view of pain due to 'wear and tear' or such simplifications. Services such as pain clinics can provide extra help for people in particular difficulty, but access to such facilities within the NHS is far less than is needed to serve the level of demand.

Chronic back pain is real but it may also be a result of underlying psychological and social stresses, some of which may not be initially apparent to either the patient or the doctor. Back pain sufferers can become disenchanted with conventional medical treatment when it fails to produce a cure. Worse is the feeling that they are not being taken seriously, are thought to be exaggerating the problem or are work-shy. Pain is sometimes a sign of internal distress from other directions and a mature medical approach to treatment will not only provide good advice and the right painkillers but will explore the background factors that can worsen or prolong the symptoms.

Key Points

- Acute back pain is one of the commonest of all problems and most episodes clear up within a few weeks.
- Keeping active is much better than prolonged rest for acute pain and simple painkillers also help.
- Sciatica is the condition in which some nerve roots are trapped by a bulging (prolapsed) disc between two vertebrae.
- Cauda equina syndrome is a rare but important complication of prolapsed disc that needs to be recognised and treated urgently.
- About one in 20 people with acute pain develop long-term back pain.
- Chronic back pain is most likely to develop in someone who has background factors such as stress or an unsatisfactory work situation.
- Successful treatment of chronic back pain is difficult in a small minority of people, who are best helped by a holistic approach from health professionals.

Appendix A

References

General

- An extensive collection of summarised references on various topics related to arthritis is on the Bandolier evidence-based medical information website at http://www.jr2.ox.ac.uk/bandolier/booth/booths/bones.html
- 'Arthritis; the big picture' (Arthritis Research Campaign); http://www.arc.org.uk/about_arth/bigpic.htm

Analgesics

- Towheed, T.E., et al., 'Analgesia and non-aspirin, non-steroidal anti-inflammatory drugs for osteoarthritis of the hip' (Cochrane Library, Issue 3, 2000); http://www.update-software.com/abstracts/ab000517.htm

- Wolfe, F., et al., 'Preference for nonsteroidal anti-inflammatory drugs over acetaminophen by rheumatic disease patients' (Arthritis & Rheumatism, 2000; 43: 378–385); http://www.ncbi.nlm.nih.gov/entrez/query.fcgi?cmd=Retrieve&db=PubMed&list_uids=10693878&dopt=Abstract
- The Oxford league table of analgesic efficacy; http://www.jr2.ox.ac.uk/bandolier/booth/painpag/Acutrev/Analgesics/lftab.html

NSAIDs

- Hernandez-Diaz, S., and Garcia Rodriguez, L.A., 'Association between nonsteroidal anti-inflammatory drugs and upper gastrointestinal tract bleeding and perforation: an overview of epidemiological studies published in the 1990s' (Archives of Internal Medicine, 2000; 160: 2093–9); http://archinte.ama-assn.org/issues/v160n14/abs/ira90047.html
- Deeks, J.J., et al., 'Efficacy, tolerability and upper gastrointestinal safety of celecoxib for treatment of osteoarthritis and rheumatoid arthritis: systematic review of randomised control trials' (British Medical Journal, 2002; 325: 619–23); http://bmj.com/cgi/content/full/325/7365/619

Osteoarthritis

- Walker-Bone, K., et al., 'Medical management of osteoarthritis' (British Medical Journal, 2000; 321: 936–40); http://bmj.com/cgi/content/full/321/7266/936
- Little, C.V., et al., 'Herbal therapy for treating osteoarthritis (Cochrane Review)' (Cochrane Library, Issue 3, 2002); http://www.update-software.com/abstracts/ab002947.htm
- Reginster, J.Y., et al., 'Long-term effects of glucosamine sulphate on osteoarthritis progression: a randomised, placebo-controlled clinical trial' (Lancet, 2001; 357: 251–6).
- McAlindon, T.E., et al., 'Glucosamine and chondroitin for treatment of osteoarthritis. A systematic quality assessment and meta-analysis' (Journal of the American Medical Association, 2000; 283: 1469–73);

http://jama.ama-assn.org/issues/v283n11/abs/jma90011.html

Rheumatoid arthritis

- Arnett, F.C., et al., 'The American Rheumatism Association 1987 revised criteria for the classification of rheumatoid arthritis' (Arthritis & Rheumatism, 1988; 31: 315–24); http://www.ncbi.nlm.nih.gov/ entrez/query.fcgi?cmd=Retrieve&db=PubMed&list_uids=3358796 &dopt=Abstract
- Uhlig, T., et al., 'Current tobacco smoking, formal education, and the risk of rheumatoid arthritis' (Journal of Rheumatology, 1999; 26(1): 1–3); http://www.ncbi.nlm.nih.gov/entrez/query.fcgi?cmd= Retrieve&db=PubMed&list_uids=9918239&dopt=Abstract
- 'Prescribing and monitoring of disease-modifying anti-rheumatic drugs for inflammatory arthritis' (Arthritis Research Campaign); http:/ /www.arc.org.uk/about_arth/med_reports/series4/ip/6508/6508.htm
- 'Guidance on the use of Etanercept and Infliximab for the treatment of rheumatoid arthritis' (National Institute for Clinical Excellence); http://www.nice.org.uk/Docref.asp?d=29671
- Gruenwald, J., et al., 'Effect of cod liver oil on symptoms of rheumatoid arthritis' (Advances in Therapeutics, 2002 Mar–Apr; 19(2): 101–7); http://www.ncbi.nlm.nih.gov/entrez/query.fcgi?cmd=Retrieve &db=PubMed&list_uids=12069368&dopt=Abstract
- Tidow-Kebritchi, S., and Mobarhan, S., 'Effects of diets containing fish oil and vitamin E on rheumatoid arthritis' (Journal of Rheumatology, 2000 Oct; 27(10): 2343–6); http://www.ncbi.nlm.nih.gov/ entrez/query.fcgi?cmd=Retrieve&db=PubMed&list_uids= 11669239&dopt=Abstract

Physiotherapy

- Welch, V., et al., 'Therapeutic ultrasound for osteoarthritis of the knee' (Cochrane Library, Issue 3, 2001); http://www.update-software.com/abstracts/ab003132.htm
- Cushnaghan, J., et al., 'Taping the patella medially: a new treatment

for osteoarthritis of the knee joint' (British Medical Journal, 1994; 308: 753–5); http://bmj.com/cgi/content/full/308/6931/753

Osteoporosis

- 'Primary Care Strategy for Osteoporosis and Falls' (National Osteoporosis Society); http://www.nos.org.uk/PDF/PCGDoc2002.pdf
- 'Osteoporosis' (Arthritis Research Campaign); http://www.arc.org.uk/about_arth/booklets/6028/6028.htm

Back Pain

- Tulder, M.W. van, et al., 'Non-steroidal anti-inflammatory drugs for low back pain (Cochrane Review)' (Cochrane Library, Issue 3, 2002); http://www.update-software.com/abstracts/ab000396.htm
- Guzmán, J., et al., 'Multidisciplinary rehabilitation for chronic low back pain: systematic review' (British Medical Journal, 2001; 322: 1511–16); http://bmj.com/cgi/content/full/322/7301/1511
- Jayson, M.I.V., 'Why does acute back pain become chronic?' (British Medical Journal, 1997; 314: 1639); http://bmj.com/cgi/content/full/314/7095/1639
- 'Back Pain' (review from the Bandolier information service); http://www.jr2.ox.ac.uk/bandolier/band19/b19-1.html
- 'Acute low back pain – management guidelines for general practitioners (2001)' (Royal College of General Practitioners); http://www.rcgp.org.uk/rcgp/clinspec/guidelines/backpain/index.asp

Hughes' syndrome

- Dr Graham Hughes, 'Hughes' syndrome. A patient's guide to the antiphospholipid syndrome'; http://www.lupus.org.uk/Publications&LUPUS.html

Drugs used in Arthritis and Rheumatic Conditions

Only brief details of each drug are given here. Full details are included in the manufacturer's data sheets and can also be viewed within the medicines section of the NetDoctor website http://www.netdoctor. co.uk/medicines/

The information is accurate at the time of writing but new information on medicines appears regularly. A health professional should always be consulted concerning the prescription and use of medicines.

Medicines and their possible side effects can affect individual people in different ways. The following lists some of the side effects that are known to be associated with these medicines. Side effects other than those listed may exist.

Painkillers

CO-DYDRAMOL
This medicine contains two active ingredients, paracetamol and dihydrocodeine.

Paracetamol is a medicine used in the treatment of mild to moderate pain. It is also useful for reducing fever. It does not reduce inflammation as well as some other pain relievers (such as aspirin or ibuprofen), but has fewer side effects than these medicines.

Dihydrocodeine belongs to a group of medicines called opioids. Opioids mimic the effects of naturally occurring pain-reducing chemicals (endorphins) found in the brain and spinal cord. They act on the opioid receptors in the brain and block the transmission of pain signals. Therefore, even though the cause of the pain may remain, the perception of the pain is changed.

Main side effects
- Headache
- Constipation
- Nausea
- Balance problems involving the inner ear (vertigo)
- Dizziness
- Hypersensitivity reactions such as narrowing of the airways (bronchospasm), swelling of the lips, throat and tongue
- Blood disorders
- Skin rashes.

How can this medicine affect other medicines?
When taken together with other medicines that have a sedative effect on the central nervous system, for example alcohol, sleeping medicines, antidepressants and antihistamines, drowsiness is likely to be increased. An excessive intake of alcohol may increase the risk of damage to the liver when taken with paracetamol. Paracetamol may increase the blood thinning effects of warfarin and other anti-coagulant medicines.

IBUPROFEN

Ibuprofen belongs to a group of medicines called non-steroidal anti-inflammatory drugs (NSAIDs). It works by blocking the action of an enzyme in the body called cyclo-oxygenase. Cyclo-oxygenase is involved in the production of various chemicals in the body, some of which are known as prostaglandins. Prostaglandins are produced in response to injury or certain diseases and would otherwise go on to cause pain, swelling and inflammation. Ibuprofen is therefore used to prevent these symptoms occurring.

Main side effects

- Headache
- Rash
- Stomach or duodenal ulcer
- Bleeding from the stomach or intestine
- Disturbances of the gut such as indigestion, diarrhoea, constipation, nausea, vomiting or abdominal pain
- Fluid retention, resulting in swelling (oedema)
- Dizziness
- Damage to the kidneys
- Blood disorders
- Liver disorders
- Allergic reactions such as skin rash, swelling of the lips, tongue and throat (angioedema) or narrowing of the airways (bronchospasm).

How can this medicine affect other medicines?

There may be an increased risk of bleeding if ibuprofen is taken with blood thinning or anti-clotting medicines such as warfarin.

There may be an increased risk of side effects such as stomach irritation if ibuprofen is taken with corticosteroids such as prednisolone.

Ibuprofen may decrease the blood pressure lowering effects of amlodipine and possibly other antihypertensive medicines.

The use of ibuprofen with diuretics, ACE inhibitors or cyclosporin may increase the risk of kidney problems.

Ibuprofen may prevent the removal of lithium and methotrexate from the body, resulting in increased blood levels of these medicines.

Ibuprofen should not be taken with any other NSAID, due to an increased risk of side effects.

Disease-modifying anti-rheumatic drugs (DMARDs)

METHOTREXATE

Methotrexate is part of a group of medicines called 'cytotoxic anti-metabolites'. It is used in the treatment of certain cancers, rheumatoid arthritis and severe psoriasis. Cancers form when some cells within the body multiply uncontrollably and abnormally. These cells then spread and destroy nearby tissues. Methotrexate acts by slowing this process down. It kills cancer cells by attaching to a chemical within the cell and preventing the cell from using vital nutrients and other substances necessary for normal cell division and activity. Methotrexate is also used in conditions where the immune system works too strongly, for example in rheumatoid arthritis and severe psoriasis. Here, the immune system attacks the body's own tissues. The precise mechanism of action of methotrexate in rheumatoid arthritis is not fully understood.

Unfortunately, methotrexate also affects the division of normal, healthy cells and therefore it produces serious side effects during high-dose, long-term treatment. The most important side effect is in the bone marrow where blood cells are made. Regular blood tests are therefore needed to monitor this effect, which is usually reversible.

Methotrexate can be taken by mouth as a tablet or be given by injection. It is recommended that effective contraceptive measures be taken when either partner is taking methotrexate.

Main side effects
- Lung disorders
- Abnormal reaction of the skin to light, usually a rash (photo-sensitivity)
- Hair loss (alopecia)
- Decreased production of blood cells by the bone marrow (bone marrow suppression)

- Damage to the liver
- Nausea and vomiting
- Damage to the kidneys
- Inflammation of the lining of the mouth (stomatitis)
- Possible decrease in fertility in both men and women.

How can this medicine affect other medicines?

This medicine decreases the body's ability to fight infections. Therefore the effectiveness of vaccines may be reduced and generalised infections may occur in individuals given live vaccines.

The following medicines may increase the risk of adverse effects of methotrexate: non-steroidal anti-inflammatory drugs (NSAIDs), retinoids, cyclosporin, probenecid and co-trimoxazole. Folic acid or folinic acid (and vitamin preparations containing these) may affect the effectiveness of methotrexate.

SULFASALAZINE

Sulfasalazine is a type of medicine called an aminosalicylate. It is used for reducing inflammation in inflammatory bowel diseases and rheumatoid arthritis. It is not fully understood how sulfasalazine works, but it is known to have antibacterial and anti-inflammatory actions. It reduces the actions of substances in the body that produce inflammation. In rheumatoid arthritis sulfasalazine reduces inflammation and damage in the joints, and therefore reduces joint swelling and stiffness. It can take up to six weeks for the full effect to be seen in rheumatoid arthritis.

Main side effects

- Difficulty in sleeping (insomnia)
- Loss of appetite
- Seizures (convulsions)
- Balance problems involving the inner ear (vertigo)
- Sensation of ringing, or other noise in the ears (tinnitus)
- Inflammation of the liver (hepatitis)
- Blood in the urine

- Inflammation of the lining of the mouth (stomatitis)
- Allergic skin reactions
- Kidney disorders
- Raised temperature
- Headache
- Rash
- Nausea
- Blood disorders
- Lung disorders
- Decreased sperm count.

How can this medicine affect other medicines?

Sulfasalazine may interfere with the absorption of digoxin or folic acid from the gut, and hence reduce their blood levels.

HYDROXYCHLOROQUINE

Hydroxychloroquine is used in the treatment of some auto-immune diseases, such as rheumatoid arthritis and systemic lupus erythematosus. It is thought to act by interfering with the production and release of blood cells that are involved in the body's immune defence system. Hydroxychloroquine is also used in treating skin conditions that are caused or aggravated by sunlight.

Main side effects

- Rash
- Blurred vision
- Changes in skin pigmentation
- Dislike of light (photophobia)
- Balance problems involving the inner ear (vertigo)
- Hair loss (alopecia)
- Disorders of the front layer of the eye (cornea)
- Worsening of the skin condition psoriasis
- Gastric disturbances including nausea, vomiting, gastric discomfort, constipation, diarrhoea

- Worsening of porphyria
- Disorder of the retina resulting in impairment or loss of vision.

How can this medicine affect other medicines?

Hydroxychloroquine may increase the blood levels of digoxin, resulting in an increased risk of side effects or toxicity. The absorption of hydroxychloroquine may be reduced by antacids (indigestion remedies), so it is advisable to leave a 4-hour interval between the two doses.

SODIUM AUROTHIOMALATE

Sodium aurothiomalate is an injectable form of the precious metal gold. It is often simply called 'Gold'. While it is not known exactly how this medicine works it is thought to damp down some elements of the body's immune response, which are indirectly responsible for the swelling, pain and inflammation of the disease. It is used in the treatment of active rheumatoid arthritis and juvenile chronic arthritis.

Main side effects
- Skin rashes
- Mouth ulcers
- Blood disorders
- Lung disorders
- Kidney disease
- Inflammation of the large intestine (colitis)
- Damage to the liver
- Loss of hair
- Skin pigmentation on areas that are exposed to sun. In long-term treatment this may be permanent.
- 'Pins and needles' sensation in hands and feet (peripheral neuritis).

How can this medicine affect other medicines?

If sodium aurothiomalate is used together with medicines that cause similar side effects, there is an increased risk of those side effects developing. This is particularly true of kidney and bone marrow problems. There is an increased risk of side effects from aspirin, phenylbutazone or oxyphenbutazone if taken together with sodium aurothiomalate.

PENICILLAMINE

It is not understood exactly how penicillamine works when used to treat rheumatoid arthritis. However, it is known that it reduces the blood levels of certain inflammatory chemicals that the body's immune system produces in rheumatoid arthritis. Once these levels have fallen, the joint symptoms subside. Penicillamine may take up to three months to work, but if it has had no effect in one year then it should be stopped.

Main side effects

- Nausea
- Blood disorders
- Skin rashes
- Lung disorders
- Kidney disease
- Abnormal enlargement of breasts in the male (gynaecomastia)
- Mouth ulcers
- Decreased appetite
- Fever
- Loss of hair
- Alteration in taste
- Chronic inflammatory disease affecting the skin and various internal organs similar to systemic lupus erythematosus (lupus syndrome).

How can this medicine affect other medicines?

Penicillamine should not be used with other medicines that reduce the ability of the bone marrow to make blood cells. This means that some of the other medicines such as gold or hydroxychloroquine used for severe arthritis should not be used at the same time as penicillamine.

INFLIXIMAB

Infliximab is a type of medicine called a monoclonal antibody. It suppresses part of the immune system and modifies the process of inflammation. It works by binding to and preventing the activity of a specific protein in the body called tumour necrosis factor alpha (TNF alpha). TNF alpha is involved in producing inflammation and controls the activity of other inflammatory chemicals.

TNF alpha is found in the joints of people with rheumatoid arthritis and in the inflamed lining of the intestine of people with Crohn's disease. Preventing the action of TNF alpha prevents the inflammatory responses it causes. Treatment with infliximab reduces infiltration of inflammatory cells into inflamed areas of the joints in rheumatoid arthritis, and into inflamed areas of the intestines in Crohn's disease. It also reduces the presence of other inflammatory markers.

Infliximab must be used in combination with methotrexate to treat rheumatoid arthritis. It is given as a drip into a vein (intravenous infusion) over a two-hour period. For rheumatoid arthritis treatment this is then repeated at two weeks and six weeks after the first infusion, then every eight weeks thereafter.

Main side effects

- Headache
- Depression
- Confusion
- Fatigue
- Agitation
- Blood disorders
- Increased tendency to infections
- Disturbances of the gut such as diarrhoea, constipation, nausea, vomiting or abdominal pain
- Abnormal heart beats (arrhythmias)
- Lupus syndrome
- Hot flushes
- Changes in blood pressure
- Difficulty in breathing

- Dizziness or loss of balance
- Chest pain
- Itchy rash (urticaria)
- Disturbances of liver function
- Pain in the muscles and joints
- Increased sweating.

How can this medicine affect other medicines?
Since infliximab is a relatively new medicine, there is insufficient information about its potential interactions with other medicines.

Drugs used in osteoporosis

ALENDRONATE
Alendronate is a type of medicine called a bisphosphonate. Bone cells continuously deposit and remove calcium and phosphorous, stored in the protein network that makes up the structure of the bone. Biphosphonates work by binding very tightly to bone, preventing the removal of calcium from the bone cells. This decreases breakdown and turnover of bone in the body and the increased calcium content leads to stronger bones. In osteoporosis, bone turnover is increased, causing the bones to become weak and prone to breaking. This medicine slows down the process of bone breakdown, so keeping bones stronger and helping to prevent fractures. It is used to treat osteoporosis and prevent fractures in people with the disease, and also to prevent bone loss in people at risk of developing osteoporosis.

Main side effects
- Headache
- Rash
- Excess gas in the stomach and intestines (flatulence)
- Disturbances of the gut such as diarrhoea, constipation, nausea, vomiting or abdominal pain
- Swelling of abdomen (abdominal distension)
- Indigestion (dyspepsia)

- Low blood calcium level (hypocalcaemia)
- Pain in muscles or bones (musculoskeletal pain)
- Flushing of the skin due to widening of the small blood vessels
- Blood in the stools
- Inflammation of the gullet (oesophagitis)
- Difficulty or pain when swallowing
- Ulceration of the gullet (oesophagus)
- Acid regurgitation
- Abnormal reaction of the skin to light, usually a rash (photosensitivity)
- Inflammation of the front parts of the eye (uveitis).

How can this medicine affect other medicines?
Calcium supplements, antacids and possibly some other medicines taken by mouth may interfere with the absorption of alendronate. For this reason one should wait at least 30 minutes after taking alendronate, before taking any other medicines by mouth.

Drugs used in gout

ALLOPURINOL
Allopurinol reduces the formation of uric acid, which is a normal by-product of the metabolism within the body of a type of protein called purine. Uric acid crystals are found within the joints and tissues in gout. By lowering the production of uric acid, gout can be prevented. Allopurinol is used for the long-term prevention of gout and not for its immediate treatment.

Uric acid is contained in some types of kidney stone and allopurinol can be used to help prevent the formation of such stones.

Main side effects
- Rash
- High blood pressure (hypertension)
- Drowsiness
- Blood disorders

- Disturbances of the gut such as diarrhoea, constipation, nausea, vomiting or abdominal pain
- Visual disturbances
- Joint pain
- Balance problems involving the inner ear (vertigo)
- Fever
- Loss of hair
- Inflammation of the liver (hepatitis)
- Alteration in taste.

How can this medicine affect other medicines?

Allopurinol increases the effects of azathioprine and mercaptopurine (cytotoxic drugs), leading to an increased risk of side effects. The side effects of ACE inhibitors and angiotensin II antagonists (drugs used mainly to treat high blood pressure) may be increased by allopurinol. Using allopurinol along with the antibiotics ampicillin or amoxycillin increases the chance of a rash developing.

Steroids

PREDNISOLONE

Prednisolone is a type of medicine known as a corticosteroid. Corticosteroids are hormones produced naturally by the adrenal glands that have many important functions, including control of inflammatory responses. Prednisolone is a synthetic corticosteroid and is used to decrease inflammation. Prednisolone works by acting within cells to prevent the release of certain chemicals that are important in the immune system. These chemicals are normally involved in producing immune and allergic responses, resulting in inflammation. By decreasing the release of these chemicals in a particular area, inflammation is reduced. This can help control a wide number of diseases characterised by excessive inflammation. They include severe allergic reactions, inflammation of the lungs in asthma and inflammation of the joints in arthritis.

Prednisolone also decreases the numbers of white blood cells circulating in the blood. This, along with the decrease in inflammatory chemicals, can prevent the rejection of organ transplants, as it prevents the body from attacking foreign tissue. It is useful for the treatment of certain types of leukaemia, where there is an abnormally large production of certain white blood cells. It is also used to treat other auto-immune diseases.

Prednisolone can be given orally or as an injection for all these purposes. It may be given by injection directly into a joint to relieve inflammation and pain and increase mobility of the affected joint, in conditions such as arthritis and tennis elbow.

Prednisolone is used in much higher doses than the levels of corticosteroids produced naturally by the body, and as such, the usual actions of corticosteroids become exaggerated and can be observed as side effects of this medicine.

Main side effects
(Most of the side effects caused by steroids increase in proportion to the dose and the length of time the drug is taken.)

- Difficulty in sleeping
- Depression
- Thinning of the skin
- Increased pressure inside the eye (glaucoma)
- Weight gain
- Irregular menstrual cycle
- Decreased functioning of the adrenal gland (adrenal suppression)
- Thinning of the bones (osteoporosis)
- Ulceration of the stomach or intestine
- Increased susceptibility to infections
- Acne
- High blood pressure (hypertension)
- Yeast infection of the moist areas of the body, especially the vagina
- Suppression of growth in children and adolescents (in high or prolonged doses).

How can this medicine affect other medicines?

The following medicines may increase the effects of corticosteroids:

- Antifungals, e.g. itraconazole and ketoconazole
- oral contraceptives.

The following medicines may increase the removal of corticosteroids from the body, thus reducing their effects:

- antiepileptics, e.g. carbamazepine and phenytoin
- barbiturates, e.g. phenobarbitone
- rifampicin.

Antacids may decrease the absorption of corticosteroids from the gut.

When taken with carbenoxolone, amphotericin or diuretics, e.g. frusemide, there is an increased risk of low blood potassium levels (hypokalaemia).

When taken with non-steroidal anti inflammatory drugs (NSAIDs), e.g. ibuprofen, there is an increased risk of adverse effects on the gut, such as stomach ulceration and bleeding.

The blood levels of salicylates, e.g. aspirin, are decreased by corticosteroids and therefore may increase to excessive levels once the corticosteroid is stopped.

Corticosteroids may oppose the treatment of high blood pressure and heart failure as they may cause retention of salt and water.

As corticosteroids may increase blood sugar, they can oppose the blood sugar lowering effects of antidiabetic medicines.

Live vaccines should not be administered to people taking corticosteroids, as their normal immune response is reduced and giving a live vaccine may therefore result in infection rather than the production of antibodies.

As corticosteroids reduce the normal response of the immune system to attack by micro-organisms, it should be ensured that if antibiotics are required, they are given in effective doses.

Appendix C

Useful Addresses

Arthritis Care

Main UK voluntary organisation for people with arthritis. Has a network of nearly 600 national branches and groups. Offers helpline support and information, a range of useful publications and self-management and personal development courses, and runs four accessible hotels.

18 Stephenson Way
London NW1 2HD
Tel: 020 7380 6500
Fax: 020 7380 6505
Website: www.arthritiscare.org.uk

Arthritis Research Campaign

Supports research and provides an extensive range of information through the website and national and local offices.

Copeman House
St Mary's Court
St Mary's Gate
Chesterfield
Derbyshire S41 7TD
Tel: 0870 850 5000 or 01246 558033
Fax: 01246 558007
Website: www.arc.org.uk

Lupus (SLE) support and information

Lupus UK
St James House
Eastern Road
Romford
Essex RM1 3NH
Tel: 01708 731251
Fax: 01708 731252
Website: www.lupusuk.com

St Thomas' Lupus Trust
The Rayne Institute
St Thomas' Hospital
London SE1 7EH
Tel: 020 7922 8197
Website: www.lupus.org.uk

Osteoporosis

National Osteoporosis Society
Camerton
Bath BA2 0PJ
Tel: 01761 471771 (general enquiries)
Helpline: 01761 472721
Fax: 01761 471104
Website: www.nos.org.uk

Psoriatic arthritis

Psoriatic Arthropathy Alliance
PO Box 111
St Albans
Herts AL2 3JQ
Tel: 0870 7703212
Fax: 0870 7703213
Website: www.paalliance.org

Homeopathy

British Homeopathic Association
15 Clerkenwell Close
London EC1R 0AA
Tel: 020 7566 7800
Fax: 020 7566 7815
Website: www.trusthomeopathy.org

Chiropractors

British Chiropractic Association
Blagrave House
17 Blagrave Street
Reading

Berkshire RG1 1QB
Tel: 0118 950 5950
Fax: 0118 958 8946
Website: www.chiropractic-uk.co.uk

Herbalists

National Institute of Medical Herbalists
56 Longbrook Street
Exeter
Devon EX4 6AH
Tel: 01392 426022
Fax: 01392 498963
Website: www.nimh.org.uk